Have Your Cake and Be Happy, Too:
A Joyful Approach to Weight Loss

Have Your Cake and Be Happy, Too:
A Joyful Approach to Weight Loss

Michelle Hastie

Absolute Love Publishing

Absolute Love Publishing

Have Your Cake and Be Happy, Too: A Joyful Approach to Weight Loss

A book by Absolute Love Publishing

Published by Absolute Love Publishing
USA

© 2017 Michelle Hastie Thompson
Photo © Pinkcandy on Shutterstock

Cover design by Logynn Hailley

United States of America

By Michelle Hastie

The Weight Loss Shift: Be More, Weigh Less

The Chakra Secret: What Your Body Is Telling You

Have Your Cake and Be Happy, Too: A Joyful Approach to Weight Loss

Dedication

I dedicate this book to my incredible little family. To Rome, the happiest, silliest little boy who has made me a proud mama for the rest of my life. To my husband, Nick, whose selflessness and kindness grants me the ability to do what I love while feeling as loved as any woman possibly can. Lastly, to Lola and Jackson, the two sweetest pit bulls who were always willing to share their love, cuddles, and kisses as I wrote this book.

Praise for Have Your Cake and Be Happy, Too

"Every so often a book is written that finally gets to the root of an issue. Michelle Hastie's *Have Your Cake and Be Happy, Too* is exactly that. Hastie not only decodes the mystery of why diet after diet seems to fail, but she also lays out her simple solution. It's an easy-to-follow method that shows you exactly how to lose weight and keep it off, WITHOUT having to deprive or starve yourself. A great read that can transform your life – I highly recommend it!" – **Alex Bratty, Online Business Strategist and Bestselling author of *From Chaos to Clarity: Getting Unstuck & Creating a Life You Love***

"This refreshing approach to weight loss is a must-read for anyone who wants to be free of dieting, shame, and guilt for good. Our minds and bodies work better when they're in sync, and Michelle shows us exactly how to stop fighting with ourselves and start living our best lives." – **Rebecca Reynandez, Founder of Spring Media Strategies**

"One of the things I've always admired about Michelle Hastie–besides her inestimable knowledge of what it *really* takes to lose weight and the crucial role of 'the inside job' that's needed to create lasting results–is her unparalleled belief in her unorthodox approach to weight loss and her faithfulness to what she knows will help people. *Have Your Cake and Be Happy, Too: A Joyful Approach to Weight Loss* is one of the best books I've read that takes an effective, holistic approach to weight loss and transforms this challenge into a joy." – **Geoff Laughton, Your Relationship Architect and author of *Building a Conflict-Proof Relationship* and *Built to Last: Designing & Maintaining a Passionate, Loving, and Lasting Relationship***

Author's Note

As a doctoral student, it is important for me to back up the theories and statements in this book with research, and you will find those sources cited. However, I have been studying psychology and weight since 2006. Along the way, I have picked up information and knowledge from credible sources that I cannot necessarily reference now, simply due to length of time. I also refer to personal experience and anecdotal evidence that is not necessarily endorsed by the natural science community. However, the scientific community has not yet studied every aspect of weight loss and psychology that I address here so I am using personal experience and anecdotal evidence where there is no hard scientific data.

Some of the information offered in this book also is intuitive. Not everything in life and weight loss can be explained scientifically, and accepting a little mystery allows me to live with infinite possibilities. I invite you to keep an open mind when reading this book, even in the instances where traditional science has yet to make an appearance. As much as I adore the process of research, I am completely open to a little "magic" as well. It is my belief that you'll go much further with your weight-loss journey if you are, too.

With Love,

Michelle

Contents

Introduction

It's a typical weekday. You wake at 6 a.m. to a blaring alarm or your son jumping on the bed, demanding breakfast. You sigh, stretch, and with a deep breath make your way out of bed—only to pass yourself in the mirror.

There it is, you think, *the 30 pounds I just can't seem to lose.*

Most days you attempt to avoid the mirror altogether, but sometimes your eyes wander, and the whirlwind of emotions begins. You think about how much you desperately want to see a different body. You focus on each perceived flaw, every roll and dimple in your skin. You imagine how a smaller, lighter body would cause all of your pain to go away, making it magically disappear along with the extra weight.

Your son interrupts your persistent thoughts.

"Cheerios! Cheerios! Cheerios!" he squeals from his place outside the door.

So you sigh again and turn from the mirror, leaving the room with a flick of the light. You walk heavily toward the kitchen, just like you did the morning before and the ones before that, all the while dreaming of an alternate body, where rolls and dimples don't exist.

Most days, you're lucky if you manage to grab a bite before piling the kids into the car and heading to school and then work. If you're feeling extra hungry, you may consider grabbing something fast: a croissant or a breakfast sandwich. A small moment of pleasure, inhaled hastily with one hand still on the wheel.

A short while later, coffee cup in hand, you push upon the door to your office. You know as long as you stay busy, you won't think about food so you do your best to fill the time. As soon as a lull hits, though, the food starts to call to you.

Just a small bite, you think. *No, don't be silly*, you immediately admonish. *I'm not hungry. I just ate.*

You try to stay focused on your work, but your brain keeps going back to food.

Maybe I am hungry, you think. *And I shouldn't deny myself if I'm hungry.* So you make your way to the kitchen.

The food goes down so quickly you barely taste the flavors, but you are aware of the momentary pleasure it brings you. It's a much deserved break. Something for you. A little reward for going to the gym last night. For being a good girl.

I deserve this, you think. And so you have some more, swallowing bite after bite of your harmless snack.

Moments later, back in your office, the reality of your "harmless snack" comes back to haunt you.

Why did I do that? you think. *What's wrong with me? Why am I so weak and pathetic?*

The heavy helping of guilt and shame comes pouring over you faster than the caloric reality of your earlier snack. You feel miserable and disappointed in yourself. And it's only 10 a.m.

Several days like this go by, until you decide you absolutely must do something about it. You must buckle down and take control of your weight. You need to control your portions. Eat healthier. Move more. Limit your sugar, carbohydrates, and calories.

That's it, you think. *I just need to put myself on a plan, and everything will be fine.*

You conveniently ignore the voice in the background that attempts to remind you that this is not the first time you have made this choice. In fact, you've "taken control of your weight" over a dozen times.

"This time will be different," you tell yourself, staring hard into the mirror. "This time I won't quit."

You nod resolutely, and pull the bathroom scale out from under the sink, placing it directly underneath the towels where you'll be sure to see it. You drag your treadmill back into the living room and empty the kitchen pantry of junk food. The food scale makes its annual appearance, and you begin to map out your meals for the week.

"I'll have a meal replacement shake for breakfast," you tell yourself, "then chicken, veggies, and brown rice for lunch, and a salad for dinner. That's doable."

And you believe it. You believe this time will be different, and you will change.

As you begin prepping your meals, your eyes wander over to your husband and your son who are eating Cheetos and laughing uncontrollably. You sigh wistfully, thinking, *I'm not lucky enough to eat Cheetos and stay thin.* And so you go back to chopping lettuce for your healthy and perfectly planned dinners, and vaguely—in the back of your mind— feel left out.

The next day, your alarm goes off at 5 a.m., an hour early. You drag your tired body over to the treadmill and get to work. *I'm doing it!* you think. *I am beating this weight thing once and for all.*

The first week is excruciating, but you manage to follow your diet and exercise routine religiously. Then, it's the moment of truth. Seven days of meal planning have passed, and you decide it's time to check your progress. The scale will tell you whether all your sacrifice was worth it. With a little apprehension and a positive mindset, you step onto the cold metal to witness all your hard work reflected back to you.

Your jaw drops. Not a pound lost. *How is that possible?* you wonder. *All that hard work ... for nothing.*

You're stunned. See, every other time you have done this— meal planned and exercised with devotion—it has worked. The scale has always moved down. Sure, the weight always came back when you get off track, but up until this this point if you followed the plan, the plan worked.

Tears begin to roll down your face. Just then, you are interrupted by two little hands wrapping around your legs.

"Whatcha doin', Mommy?"

And so you wipe your tears, pick up your son, and start preparing dinner for your family. But you can't get rid of the disappointment, the frustration, the hopelessness of ever achieving the body you desire so deeply.

Countless people embark on this journey every year, and most of them believe—just as you have believed—that they fail. They believe that if they don't lose weight, or if they gain the weight back, there is something wrong with them, not the method.

But that belief is mistaken. You, and they, didn't fail. **The method failed.**

There is something fundamentally wrong with traditional weight-loss methods. They require you to put your life on hold while you attempt to achieve your ideal body. They convince you that temporary suffering is necessary to get what you want. They make it impossible to achieve success.

With traditional weight-loss methods, it is normal to feel like quitting, to feel deprived, to feel punished for putting on extra pounds when you should have known better. But there is another way. A better way.

Instead of asking you to put your life on hold, this way asks you to lose weight while living your life. In fact, **this method of weight loss requires you to be so incredibly full of life that your body has no choice but to transform.** Of course there are steps you will take to help your body transform, but they add to your life instead of take away from it.

And you can lose weight this way. Anybody can. It simply involves a new way of looking at food, exercise, your body, and your life. It requires you to give up your current reality and commit to living your dream life. The one that feels impossible to live right now.

This way also requires that you learn to live the way naturally thin people live. See, naturally thin people—the people who don't fear weight gain, who eat what they want and move when they want—are doing things differently than you. And most of them aren't even aware of it. It's automatic, just like the things you and other chronic dieters are doing automatically that keep weight on your body. And these automatic processes and perspectives are why you believe you have failed over and over again using traditional weight-loss methods.

Are you ready for a better way?

What Does It Mean to Lose Weight While Living Your Life?

This book is based on the premise that you can lose weight while you live your life. That you don't have to put anything on hold to succeed. That you don't have to suffer to have the body you desire.

Other methods of weight loss require that you utilize external methods to remove your weight. They ask you to disconnect and ignore the body. They tell you not to trust your cravings, your appetite, or your body in general. They convince you that you can be smarter than your body, as if your intellect can win over the perfectly designed and incredibly complex machine that is your body.

Your body is amazing. It can mend broken bones and heal open wounds. It can digest food, eliminating what it doesn't need and utilizing what it does. It keeps your heart beating and regulates its own temperature without any direction from you. It protects itself from toxins and chemicals and has an entire army ready to fight foreign invaders at the drop of a hat.

It also releases fat it doesn't need. It does this flawlessly, naturally. It's not something you need to interfere with or learn how to do. You just need to learn how to connect with your body so you can best support it in its weight-loss process.

This is not typical weight loss talk. Traditional weight-loss methods want you to subdue your body. To conquer it. But you are not meant to conquer your body. That will not, and does not, support your goals.

You are the nurse to your body, not the drill sergeant. Your job is to ask it what it needs and nurse it to optimum health. And this doesn't require much of your energy. It is not an around-the-clock, 24/7 obligation. A simple check-in here and there to see what the body needs and then an effort to provide it is all that is required. Then you can go back to living your life.

Your body is designed to do the heavy lifting for you. It wants you to focus on living, not losing. When you do, you will reap the benefits you so desperately desire.

How do I know this? I have practiced it. I have learned it. Better still, I have had the incredible blessing to be able to teach my clients these lessons and to watch them transform, just as I did.

No, I am not some type of magical creature that knows something different about my body. I have just learned the skills to best support my body in doing all the incredible things it knows how to do. Then I spend the other 23 hours of my day living—really living.

That's the best part of this method. When you focus on living from within, you have your weight-loss tools for life. They always are inside of you. It's not a matter of following someone else's diet or a meticulously plotted exercise and meal plan. It's about allowing your body's innate, perfectly designed plan to play out optimally.

And, unlike traditional weight-loss methods, this approach works. I've seen it in my own life and in the lives of the women I've coached. It's also backed by research, including the research I personally conducted for my academic thesis, "The Truth Behind Women and Weight."

As part of my research, I interviewed 42 women to investigate their beliefs, thought patterns, and behaviors around food, exercise, and weight. I wanted to see if there was a difference between those who identified as being at their "ideal weight" and those who said they were overweight. There was. The 16 women in my research group who lived at their ideal weight had an astonishingly different mindset than the 26 women in the group who felt they were too heavy.

This research supported what I already believed: External methods of weight loss nearly always fail eventually. In fact, multiple studies show that about 80 percent of dieters regain lost weight, generally within six years. The 20 percent who manage to keep the weight off don't fare much better. Research indicates that even though they don't regain the weight these 20 percent continue to fear weight gain, living lives of restriction; deprivation; and constant focus on food, exercise, and weight.

When you're a chronic dieter using traditional weight-loss methods, you remain a person with excess weight *even when you lose the weight*. In your mind, you are still someone who can't eat Cheetos and stay thin. You are still "unlucky," with "poor metabolism." You still have to watch what you eat and exercise more than your naturally thin friends.

Traditional weight-loss methods teach you that you don't have the luxury of being free with food and movement. You decide that in order to stay thin you must stay focused, even obsessed. You believe that thin, to you, will never be effortless.

And so, when you are able to trick your body into getting smaller through external methods, you find it doesn't last. It may take months. It may take years. But the weight always comes back. This is because the body always seeks to match the outside with the inside. This is likely why a 2012 study of identical twins showed that those who dieted gained more weight than their non-dieting twins.

On the inside, the dieting twin is still a person who struggles with weight so she remains a person who struggles with weight on the outside as well. Traditional weight-loss methods alter your mindset and your actions in a negative way. They perpetuate the weight loss/gain cycle, and so it continues—until you decide to try something different.

What Does It Feel Like to Lose Weight While Living Your Life?

Imagine you have decided to lose weight. This time, however, you are not going to restrict food and/or force exercise. You are going to lovingly step inside of your body and communicate with the deepest version of yourself. You become an expert not in nutrition or exercise, but in you and your body.

You learn what gives you energy and what robs it. You learn to identify your basic needs, how to take care of yourself the same way you do your loved ones. You learn what foods make you feel good and which ones don't. You find the movements that you love and crave, and you eliminate all the others.

You step out of your comfort zone and go after what you truly want. You settle for nothing less than everything you truly desire. If you can think it, you know it's possible, and you search for solutions until you get what you want.

You realize that living naturally thin is simply a skillset. It's something you can learn, practice, and master. There is no difference between you and the thin person who doesn't fear weight gain except that she has already mastered that skillset. Just as you can learn piano, you can learn how to live in a body without fear of weight. It's not saved for the lucky few. It's available to every person on the planet.

You know this now, and as a result of practicing this skillset and living the life of your dreams, your body easily releases the excess weight. There's no reason to hold onto it any longer. You master living naturally thin, and your body takes on its ideal form forever.

What Will Losing Weight While Living Your Life Do for You?

When you release the mindset learned from traditional weight-loss methods and embrace this new perspective, you will lose weight. More importantly, you will eliminate food obsessions and the fear of weight gain—forever. You will no longer have to rely on any other person or any external program to give you the body or the lifestyle you want. You will live intuitively, joyfully, and in the body you most desire.

This method is unlike any other weight-loss program. It is

more than a lifestyle change; it's an internal shift. It's mastery. With this method, you will have such massive shifts internally that you will never have to think about your weight again.

This method is more than just a set of steps to master to lose weight. Not all thin people have mastered all of these steps. The majority of thin people have mastered a few of these steps that will be outlined in the following chapters, but not all have mastered enough to live a truly free life forever. And that's what this method is: A way to lose weight and live your most incredible life.

Because the truth is not all thin people are happy. Not all thin people are living in the ways that I recommend to you. But I see more than just a smaller version of your body. I see the possibility of your dream life. And so I invite you to do more than the minimum needed to lose weight.

Become thinner yes, but do more, too. Decide you will no longer tolerate settling. Because the truth is this: You've been lying to yourself about your life.

You've convinced yourself that never achieving your desire is okay. That things could be worse. That there's no need to rock the boat.

You've convinced yourself that the life you have today isn't so bad. And there would be nothing wrong with that if your desires didn't flicker across your consciousness here and there. It would be okay if you didn't want more, but you do. You *do* want more. Sometimes you even allow yourself to dream about that "more," indulging in thoughts about all you would like to have, categorizing them as "nice-to-haves."

You've removed the urgency to live the life that you actually desire to live. You've tried too many times. You're tired. You're defeated. Your weight is one essential aspect of this mindset, but in reality there is so much more. This perspective has invaded every area of your life. It impacts your body, your mind, your career, and your relationships.

Here, today, I invite you to push through it. You *have* to push through it. You have to settle for nothing less than everything you want.

I will help you.

There are seven steps to master to live your best life in your best body. Within these pages, I will explain the minimum steps to take for **total body transformation** and then expand those steps for **total life transformation**, enabling you to live the kind of life I know you want to live. I will do my best to make this book your go-to guide to live naturally thin and to help you learn, practice, and master the art of living without fear of weight. Some people, however, may want additional contact and support.

If that's you, I am available to walk the journey with you. I've been where you are, and I've come out the other side. I've also helped countless others walk the path before you. If you want maximum support and human-to-human contact, simply fill out an application at totalbodyhealthsolutions.com/getsupport. If you qualify, I will personally get on the phone with you and help guide you through this process.

Are you ready to change your life? Let's dive in!

The Seven Steps

Live connectedly
Live intentionally
Live joyously
Live truthfully
Live abundantly
Live deliciously
Live fully

These seven steps will set up your most incredible life and

your ideal body. However, the journey is never over. The secret to living in your best body and your ideal life is to continually grow in each of these seven steps and to stay present. Presence is the effort that is required of you throughout this journey and throughout your life.

Connect with your body, with people, and the world as a whole. This connection is the key to mastering your best body on the inside first.

Bring intention to each day, and challenge yourself to notice your limiting language. Living intentionally removes limitations so your body can operate at its optimum level.

Allow joy to pour in through new and different avenues, and settle for nothing less than truthful living. Because without joy, why even be thin?

Allow abundance and deliciousness to seep in through every corner, allowing each year to bring ever more. A life with abundance and deliciousness gives your body the tools it needs to thrive.

Lastly, live a full life. Make your life so full that you have no reason to fill it with food unless you're physically hungry. Make it so fulfilling that you have no time to devote to a less-than-ideal body. If you do that, your body has no choice but to support you on your mission to live optimally.

These seven steps can be applied to every area of your life, and they can be continuously mastered. This is a good thing, because the path of achieving mastery over these steps is the true "good life." Walking the path *is* living, and—done fully—there is absolutely nothing better.

Live Connectedly

As human beings we have an innate desire to connect—with each other, with something bigger than us, and with ourselves. Unfortunately, most people who decide to lose weight do so utilizing an external method that comes with a serious consequence: It causes a disconnection between the mind and the body. This threatens the inner connection we desire so greatly.

When we are connected to ourselves and the body says it's hungry, we feed it what it wants. When the body says it is full, we stop eating. When the body says it wants to move, we move in the way we innately know will feel best. When it says it needs rest, we rest—without guilt or shame because we know it is what we need.

When we are disconnected from ourselves, however, and the body says it is hungry, we stop to calculate whether we have enough calories left in our daily allotment to feed it. Or we choose a food based on what someone else told us to eat, rather than what our body says it needs. When we are disconnected, and the body says it's full, we look down to see if there is food remaining on the plate, or we may be so disconnected that we don't even notice the fullness signal. When we are disconnected and the body says it wants to move, we move in the way outside sources have told us to move rather than in the way our body says would feel best. When the body asks for rest, we check the scale to see if we are allowed to take a rest day.

This disconnection affects us deeply. When we continually override the body, we teach the body that we don't need it. To make matters worse, we often then become angry with the body for not performing optimally for us, even though we haven't given it the attention it deserves.

We pick and pinch the body and tell it that it's not good enough. We tell it that it should digest better, metabolize faster, move better, pump blood faster, and not tire as easily. We tax our bodies, disconnect from them, and then expect them to have no reaction to this mistreatment. We beat them up at the gym and rob them of food groups, and then ask them to deal with it.

In order to live in the ideal version of the body permanently, we must first connect with the body and figure out what it needs. This is similar to what we would do when dealing with a troubled child. If a child were struggling, we wouldn't beat the child up or tell her to figure it out. We would attempt to connect to the child and find out what the child needs to succeed. This is your job with this step—connect with your body and figure out what it needs.

Naturally thin people are connected to their bodies. They eat when they are hungry. They stop when they are full. They listen to what their bodies need, and they know what they want to eat when hunger strikes. They eat that food and move on with their day, with no lingering cravings and no guilt.

This connection extends to exercise as well. Naturally thin people work out when they want and relax when that sounds better. Movement is natural and fun, not forced or punishing.

This mind-body connection allows the body to relax. Knowing that it will be taken care of, the body is able to move its focus from survival to what it does best. It digests a little better, metabolizes a little faster, and overall performs more optimally.

When we are disconnected from the body, however, we live constantly in survival mode, which means the body can never relax. Instead, it stays on high alert, scared that the resources it needs to survive will be depleted. From this fear of never having enough, the body decides to prolong what it already has, which makes everything slow down. Metabolism slows. Energy decreases. And motivation to move or change plummets.

Unfortunately for the many chronic dieters in the world, traditional weight loss methods sever the mind-body connection and thrust the body into survival mode. They teach you to not eat when you're hungry or to not eat the nutrients and ingredients your body is telling you it needs. They teach you to push yourself when your body needs to rest or to do activities that do not give your body the movement it wants. As a result, you eat carrots when you're craving meat and you run when your body wants to meditate with yoga. From this, your body learns you will not listen to its signals.

The first step to living fully while losing weight, then, is to shift from living from a place of disconnection to living from a place of full connection. You can do this through awareness and curiosity.

Many of us understand intellectually that we should be more aware of where we are in life, but most people aren't really sure how to do that. This book breaks down awareness into three easy-to-implement sections: awareness in life, awareness with food, and awareness with exercise.

With awareness comes an honest understanding of exactly where we are. In order to travel to New York by car, we must first know the state in which we're starting. If we are starting in California, we know we'll need to drive east. If we are starting in Maine, we'll need to travel south. Being aware of these differences is essential for optimal results.

Imagine, then, if you had no idea where you were and just started driving. Perhaps you were in California and chose to go south. Before long, you would reach the border and find yourself in an entirely different country.

And maybe you'd never heard of Mexico. Maybe you had no idea where you were. You only knew you were even farther away from New York than when you'd started. So you decide you must randomly choose another direction, and you hope for the best.

That's what it is like when we move forward in life without awareness. We are just like the lost traveler with a destination in mind. We know where we want to go, but we can't pinpoint where we're starting. So we just begin moving in random directions and our results are sporadic at best.

To live with awareness, you must first figure out where you are. Not where someone told you you are, or where you are pretending you are. You must actually step into your current reality and face it. It may be uncomfortable, but it is the only way you'll get a starting point from which to draw an accurate map to your ultimate destination.

Step One: Awareness in Life

Becoming present and aware in life requires you to get to know yourself. Your personality, motivations, past experiences, habits, thought processes, and emotions are all responsible for creating the person you are right in this moment. Before you begin choosing action steps toward weight loss, it is imperative that you understand yourself. Everything that makes up who you are has created this moment right now, so why are you here?

Do you hesitate to take action unless there is a guarantee?

Or are you a risk taker who is willing to try anything even if it fails?

Do you procrastinate until it becomes so uncomfortable you can't stand it? Or do you act instinctively without thinking too hard about it?

Is your toleration ceiling so high that you are willing to settle for a life less than what you truly desire? Or are you willing to settle for nothing less than everything you want?

Are you often pessimistic and don't believe you will ever truly have what you want? Or are you an optimist that expects the best?

Do you require social approval and put more weight on others' opinions than your own? Or do you put more emphasis on what you think and feel?

Try not to judge your answers to these questions. The point is not to judge. The point is to paint an accurate picture of who you are so that you can begin making changes. This is the time to get honest. What are your strengths, and what are your weaknesses? What parts of who you are today need to change in order to set yourself up for success?

Total Body Transformation:

If you're looking to transform your body, all you have to do is look in the mirror each day and acknowledge exactly where you are. When negative emotions come up, acknowledge them and then remind yourself they are simply feelings and do not have to interfere with your body's ability to lose weight. State them accurately, as feelings not life sentences, and then continue on with your day, focused on living. Bottom line: Stay present, as much as humanly possible.

Total Life Transformation:

If you want to transform more than your body, you'll need to dig deeper. Think back to the very first time you looked in the mirror and thought, *I need to lose weight.* When was it?

Often, when I ask this question, I hear answers like, "My whole life," and "Since I was born." But no one woke up as a one-year-old child thinking, *Man, I look fat today!* That thought came at some later point in your life—even if it was very early.

Find that first memory of your brain feeding you negative information about your body. You don't need to relive those emotions, but go back and look at what was going on. Did your family, friends, or a doctor say that you had a weight challenge? Was it your idea based on the bodies that were around you?

Maybe you put on weight at a certain time in your life. Dig deep into your memories of what your life looked like at the time you first remember having a weight challenge. What was going on at that time? Was being overweight your thought or somebody else's?

After you pinpoint that moment, follow it up to the present. What diets have you tried? Did they work? Which ones worked? When they worked, what was going on in your life? Were there times in your life when weight came off without you understanding why? Were there times when you were heavier, and you didn't know why? Don't worry if you don't have all of the answers. Simply ask the questions, and begin to take an inventory.

It is important to dig deeply because you'll find that we don't gain weight by accident. It's for a very specific reason or, sometimes, various reasons. Excess weight is our body's attempt to communicate with us or teach us something.

Think back to a time you had a challenge in your life and

you overcame it. Maybe you had a setback at work or lost a friend. What happened in the aftermath of that challenge? What did you do differently? What lesson did you learn? I subscribe to the idea that there is always a lesson.

We learn from our mistakes, and then we grow and move on. If we don't learn, often times we don't grow. This same process needs to happen with your body.

If you are wondering why you have never been able to keep off weight, ask yourself if you have ever stopped to learn what your body is attempting to teach you about your life. If you aren't sure, it may not be a coincidence that the extra pounds don't stay off.

Our bodies are intelligent, and they will sometimes give us weight as an indication that we need to change something about our lives, something that isn't serving us. If you don't look to heal what isn't serving you and to follow your best possible life path, your body will continue to communicate with you the only way it knows how—through your weight.

This happens for various reasons, and it is unique to each individual. A past client we will call Jessie had taken on the caregiver role for her elderly mother. She felt stretched thin and put herself last on the list each day. Through our work together, she learned to make time for herself and to let go of the unnecessary burdens she was carrying. She claims that she had to first lose 100 pounds of mental and emotional weight before her body was willing to release the physical pounds. And it did.

Like Jessie, many of us are holding onto burdens, but some are emotional: guilt, anger, fear, or sadness. Turns out, studies show that we not only hold onto these feeling emotionally, we hold onto them physically as well. The feelings can manifest as excess weight, and those around us can see it, which makes us feel ashamed. Then, because we are ashamed, we become angry with ourselves. We become mad for being where we are, and we don't know how to forgive ourselves. And this inability to forgive traps us.

You cannot move forward until you forgive yourself.

Weight can feel like a very heavy burden to carry. It feels like something you did to yourself because of bad choices in the past, though this often isn't true. When I held onto excess weight, I was doing all the "right" things. I ate healthy foods within my calorie range, and I worked out every single day. I challenged my body in and out of the gym and gave it every available tool to lose weight, yet it didn't. So even if you made the right choices, there is no guarantee that your body would be ideal for you.

It's time to forgive yourself for being where you are. If you need help with this, it may be beneficial to remember the truth behind dieting—it isn't *supposed* to work.

Diets can teach you portion control, calorie counting, meal planning, and even exercise routines, but they won't teach you life lessons, presence, or the reasons that you gained that weight in the first place. They can't. Diets are for the masses, and mass approaches don't work long-term for everyone.

In our hearts, we all know this.

When I asked participants in my research whether dieting worked, the majority said no in some way or another. Three out of four participants (76 percent) chose a response that indicated they believed dieting is ineffective in terms of the ability to lose pounds. Nineteen percent believed it could work to lose pounds, as long as a person maintains the diet for life. Less than one percent of participants said that dieting to lose weight makes you healthier.

Also, 41 percent of dieters reported gaining back any weight lost on a diet within six months or less. Thirty-eight percent were able to keep weight off for up to two years. Only two percent were able to keep the weight off for longer than two years. The majority of participants (70 percent) also reported negative side effects from dieting, and nearly nine out of 10 participants (86 percent) said they felt defeated, terrified, and/or guilty after dieting.

So be happy dieting didn't work for you. Had you been one of the few for whom it did, my research indicates that you would have had to be on that diet forever in order to keep the weight off and feel good about yourself. And who wants to live like that? Not me.

Naturally thin people don't diet. Up to the age of 21, I didn't even know what calories were. I was shocked that people counted them to monitor their body and felt ignorant that I hadn't done the same.

"How am I thin?" I asked myself. "I have no idea how many calories I eat!" It didn't occur to me at the time that the very reason I was thin was because I was blissfully unaware of the life dieters lived.

Dieting does not work. So forgive yourself for being where you are.

Stop thinking, *I can't believe I'm so big.* Stop asking, "How did I dare to allow myself to get to this place?" Stop berating yourself, thinking you don't have willpower.

You are in the exact place you are supposed to be with what you know. So give up those old stories now.

You are now getting the information you need to move forward and not battle weight. You are opening up your mind to learning more about your body. Be happy and proud that you continue to invest in yourself and are looking for solutions.

If you have tried every diet under the sun, congratulations! You are a fighter, and you refuse to give up. That is an admirable quality. It's not your fault you haven't found the right path for you. Be happy that you have the will to keep searching.

Questions for Transformation:

1. **When was the very first time I gained weight?** Pay attention to what emotions come up when you answer this question. If the first time was when you were a child, try to imagine the child version of yourself and think about what this child was thinking and feeling. Was it really your idea that you were overweight? If your weight gain was later in life, think about what else was going on at that time. Were you extra stressed? Overwhelmed? Or can you remember someone telling you that weight gain happens at this specific time?

2. **Why do I believe I gained weight at that time?** Stay out of judgment here. If you had to dig deep into the why behind your weight, what is it really about? If you have been eating too much, think about why you might be eating too much. If you are moving too little, why are you making that choice? The answers to these questions are deeper than "I am weak or lack willpower." Get curious.

3. **What gift is my weight giving me?** What could you be gaining from the process of gaining and losing weight? What challenges in the past have gifted you incredible insights for which you are forever grateful?

4. **What is the lesson I am supposed to learn from my weight gain?** If your weight could talk to you, what would it say? Would it ask for more love and acceptance? Would it ask for relaxation? Would it ask for more fun and creativity? Higher-quality food? Emotional protection?

Step Two: Awareness with Food

Total Body Transformation:

In order to transform your body, you must eat when you

are hungry and stop when you are full. This will take time to master, but you don't have to be perfect at it for it to work. Start by tweaking your current eating habits. For *at least* seven days do the following to get back in touch with hunger and fullness:

1. Each time you get the desire to eat, ask yourself, "Am I hungry?" If yes, ask yourself, "What do I want to eat?" Then eat that food.

If you don't know what food to eat, know this is normal. Just make your best guess. You can't be wrong. If anything, you may simply notice that your choice leaves you with unpleasant consequences (upset stomach, sluggishness, heartburn, etc.) In that case, you can use the information to make a different decision in the future.

If the answer is no, ask yourself, "What do I want or need?" Then choose to fulfill that want or need, even if the answer is "to eat." Sometimes we can acknowledge that we are not hungry, and we still choose to eat. This will happen less and less as you practice this technique. But in the beginning, you simply need to do what you choose to do with full awareness and without judgment.

2. If you are not noticing hunger signals, set your alarm for every three to four hours. When the alarm goes off, go through the questions above to see if you are hungry. Once you find your meal rhythm you can turn off the alarm.

3. Eat without distractions (driving, TV, computer, phone, etc.) This is essential to learning to stop when you are full. To start, take five to 10 deep breaths before putting food into your mouth, and again periodically throughout the meal to see if you're full. Eat slowly and with full awareness. As you eat, keep asking yourself, "Am I full?" At first, it might be helpful to set a certain amount of bites after which to take three deep breaths and ask this question.

Total Life Transformation:

If you want to transform more than your body and experience life at its fullest, you'll need to bring a deeper level of awareness to your eating habits. Breathing deeply is a crucial part of this awareness. Breathing gives the body time to acknowledge and taste the food we are eating so that we feel satisfied and nourished. It gives us the present state of mind to notice when we are full, and it relaxes the body, which is absolutely vital to digestion.

Picture your favorite piece of cake in front of you. It's on a delicate white plate, adorned by an artistic drizzle of raspberry or chocolate sauce. It looks delicious, and your mouth waters in preparation for your first bite. Before you pick up your fork, stop.

Get focused on your breath. Close your eyes, and take five to 10 deep breaths. Inhale deeply, and smell your cake. Keep breathing. Open your eyes, and fully experience the colors and arrangement of this perfectly cooked and plated dessert.

Take the first bite. As you chew your delectable cake, take another deep breath and put the fork down. Revel in the flavors and the textures of this favorite food of yours.

Be fully present with this piece of cake. Honor the moment and how much time and energy went into preparing your tasty treat. Don't multi-task. Be fully engaged in eating. Eat calmly, slowly, and as stress-free as possible. This speeds up your metabolism by creating an ideal environment for digestion and ensures you don't miss your body's signals that it is full.

Try to think only positive thoughts while eating. Avoid thinking, *I shouldn't be eating this cake.* Your perceptions about what you eat directly affect your digestion and metabolism.

This may sound farfetched, but science supports it. In fact, there was an interesting study done in which researchers gave participants two identical milkshakes with different labels and measured the results. One label identified the milkshake as indulgent and high-fat, while the other label identified the milkshake as low-calorie and guilt-free. Participants experienced a spike in ghrelin (a hunger hormone) when they drank the one with the high-fat label but not when they drank the low-calorie one. This study is a perfect example that what you perceive about your food has a direct correlation to what your body does in response to it.

To your body, eating when you're upset translates into being attacked by wolves. Your body reacts to negative thoughts and stress in the same way it does to danger. If you feel guilty, ashamed, unworthy, etc., your digestion and metabolism will be less optimal.

Naturally thin people have an advantage here because they don't have the emotions around food that dieters do. They simply view food as food, not the cause of everything they hate (excess weight). Awareness of your judgments and emotions around food are a necessary part of changing this process.

In my research, the ideal-weight participants described their appetites as something that felt natural, and they chose their foods for positive reasons. They also described food as pleasurable and enjoyable. The overweight participants described their appetites as out of control, and they chose their foods based on a number of things, including diet restrictions. They also described food as something that causes emotional distress.

To bring yourself closer to your ideal weight, you must change the way you view and eat food. Slow down, get aware, and leave that stress behind while you eat. For example, if you are stressed about paying a bill, be honest with yourself about the emotion. Do something about it if you can. If there is nothing you can do about it at the moment, let go of the thought, focus on your food, and get the nourishment your body needs. After a calm and fulfilling meal, you then can begin brainstorming about ways to pay that bill.

Awareness with food also means that you fully enjoy your food. Learn to be the slowest eater at the table. Take in every flavor, herb, and spice. Make mealtime a positive experience. Savor, don't just swallow.

Food awareness doesn't end with mealtime, however. You must listen, too, to what happens in your body before and after you eat. Before the meal, look at what emotions may be triggering your desire to eat particular foods. Consider whether that's really the food you want to eat, or if your desire may be coming from feelings you're experiencing around something else in your life.

A study conducted just a few years ago tested whether or not mood influences food preference. The results indicated that negative mood cues cause us to search for indulgent foods while positive mood cues lead us to search for healthy foods. This link between food and mood means it is imperative that you pay attention to how you are feeling and how food is making you feel. Bring awareness to all stages of the eating process to ensure your mind and body are connected and honoring each other.

After the meal, notice if the food you just ate actually served you. Learn to recognize connections between symptoms and food. What happens in your body after you eat a lot of dairy? Do you have stomach pain or do you feel great? What about when you eat a lot of processed foods? How do you feel afterward? Do you feel sleepy or stuffed up? Do you feel energized and fabulous?

That reciprocal honor is important. So far, we've talked about how mental awareness with food can nourish the body. But the body must also nourish the mind. Otherwise, we feel deprived and are driven to overeat or engage in other unhealthy behaviors.

If you want to live your fullest life, you must address the common problems many of us experience around food: overeating, binge eating, and starvation. In our society, we hear most about overeating. We have Overeaters Anonymous, countless weight-loss classes, and numerous books and programs that talk about weight or portion control. We are bombarded with experts who talk about how to stop binging and cope with emotional eating. But I feel that people are still missing the mark when it comes to this ever-popular topic.

From my experience working with clients and researching weight loss, I've realized that overeating has nothing to do with food. Does that statement surprise you? It's true. Overeating is not about *what* you are eating. It's about *who you are when you are eating.*

A recent study done by Kersten and Scherwitz found that overeating is a blend of "food-related eating behaviors, emotions, beliefs, habits, thoughts, sensations, environments, and social behaviors." Note that there is not a mention of genetics or personality, as many people may assume. I have found the most common causes of overeating to be lack of awareness, a fear of deprivation ("If I don't eat it all I will be deprived"), and insufficient fulfillment or satisfaction (meaning you wanted a hamburger but got a salad instead).

When we continue to eat after our stomachs are full, we jump to the conclusion that this is because we lack willpower, are pathetically greedy, or are simply addicted to food. This couldn't be further from the truth. What is really happening is that our minds are quite literally *not full.*

When we eat without awareness, our bodies get full but our minds don't feel fulfillment, satisfaction, or pleasure. This lack of satiety triggers us to search for more and more food until our *minds* finally feel full. This happens frequently when we eat something other than we're craving. If we are craving something salty, for instance, and we eat carrots instead, we likely won't feel full no matter how many carrots we eat. If we then eat a salad because we're still not satisfied, it isn't likely to help. We're still going to feel hungry, because we're still missing the thing we craved. No matter how much you eat, if you aren't eating with awareness, your mind will tell you to keep eating until *it* feels mentally and emotionally full and satisfied.

This is also true if your life doesn't feel full. If your life isn't fulfilling, satisfying, or nourishing, you will search for food to fill you up. This could come from not having the job you want or the relationship you want. When you feel empty, your mind looks for the obvious filler: food.

For some people, simply bringing presence to the meal is enough to eliminate emotional eating behaviors altogether. Make a pact with yourself to always eat with presence—not as you're walking through the house, driving your car, or watching television at the end of a hard day. Once you eliminate mindlessness around food, you'll find that binge eating stops, overeating subsides, and eating within hunger becomes simple.

Many of us also eat when we are bored. Maybe it's Sunday, and there is nothing to do, so you eat, or maybe you don't have any hobbies so you fill your time with eating. When we are lacking fun and creativity in our lives, our minds search for something obvious to fill the void.

To help address this common problem, look for ways to make your life more fun and more fulfilling. When I struggled with my weight, I often was literally and emotionally filling all the missing gaps in myself with food. It wasn't until I decided to find and follow my true life path, my career, that I completely stopped doing that.

Binge eating is a more exaggerated version of overeating that comes from a deeper, unconscious level. What's interesting about binge eating is that it is often dependent on a self-diagnosis. Johnson et al. conducted a study to compare binge eaters with non-binge eaters, and the self-proclaimed binge eaters were rarely identified as such by the judges evaluating the eating episodes. The study concluded that binge eating relies on perception, specifically the individual's feeling of being out of control. That feeling is a *subjective* experience that occurs in the mind—not the body.

Marc David, the founder of The Institute for the Psychology of Eating, claims that binge eating comes from tight control somewhere else in life. He states that if everything in our lives is very controlled (as with, for example, calorie restriction), then it's only natural that we will seek something that is out of control. I found this to be true for myself; when I stopped dieting (and thus trying to strictly control my food), I immediately stopped bingeing, too.

Some people also binge eat due to perfectionism or because they have emotions they don't know how to face. When we binge, we check out. We become numb and actually abandon consciousness. This is comforting because it keeps us from having to deal with unresolved or difficult emotions. Afterward, this comfort continues because we concentrate on feeling guilty about our bingeing instead of that other feeling, the really important one that our body wants us to experience. That feeling is camouflaged and lost.

If you find that you binge eat on a regular basis, ask yourself whether you're experiencing strict control elsewhere in your life. Are you striving too hard to be "perfect"? Are you restricting yourself too much? If not, is there anything you aren't facing, an emotion you are trying to hide?

Remember to eat, too. If you are starving yourself throughout the day, you will likely binge or overeat at night. Your body is only doing what's natural—making sure it is fed. Anytime you go too long between meals (more than four or five hours), your body believes it must binge to survive. It's as if it awoke after a long snowy winter; it will eat all it can to stay alive.

The food inventory exercise below also can help bring additional awareness to the type of eater you are. For *at least* seven days write out the following for each meal: how long it took you to eat it, how much pleasure you received from it, and how full you are.

For pleasure, you are looking for anything *above* a seven. For fullness, however, seven is optimal. Anything higher indicates that you have moved past fullness into overly full, with 10 being sick to your stomach from too much food. It is extremely important that you do not write down *what* you ate. Noting food types is a dieting strategy and not one that is of importance to us. With this exercise, we just want to find out what type of eater you are.

Food Inventory

Breakfast

Time taken to eat:
Pleasure (1—10):
Fullness (1—10):

Lunch

Time taken to eat:
Pleasure (1—10):
Fullness (1—10):

Dinner

Time taken to eat:
Pleasure (1—10):
Fullness (1—10):

Step Three: Awareness with Exercise

Total Body Transformation:

Don't live a sedentary lifestyle. If you want to transform your body, the majority of your life needs to consist of more than sitting/lying down. If each day you wake up and sit down, drive somewhere to sit down, drive home to sit down, and then fall asleep each night, you will need to move more.

If you move more than that, you don't need to make any changes with movement. It is important to point out that we are looking at the majority of time. In other words, if you go on vacation and lie by the pool, this does not mean you gain weight. If you are injured and cannot move, this does not mean you gain weight.

The question is simply, "Am I sedentary for the majority of my life?" If yes, move a little each day. That's all it takes.

Total Life Transformation:

If you want to do more than transform your body and live your ideal, fullest life, then you must re-establish the connection between your body and your mind in regard to movement just as you did with food. How do you feel when you do or do not exercise? Do you feel great every time you go to the gym? Do you get an exercise high? Do you feel exhausted and defeated? Embarrassed and out of place? What is your exercise experience doing for you?

If you have been over exercising, doing nothing may feel really good. It probably feels amazing just to sit and watch TV with no expectations of working out, or maybe doing nothing feels so foreign and dangerous that you hate it. Maybe stillness is so out of the ordinary that it feels uncomfortable. Begin to notice how you feel with and without exercise.

An interesting finding in my research was that almost all of the participants, both ideal weight and overweight, exercised at least two times per week. And although the ideal-weight participants did state they worked out daily more often than the overweight participants, it's not as if the overweight participants didn't work out at all. And yet, the resounding majority of overweight participants felt they were coming up short when it came to exercise. They felt they were not doing enough. The ideal-weight participants, on the other hand, felt they exercised a sufficient amount.

The motivation to exercise differed between the two groups, as well. The ideal-weight participants felt motivated by health and wellbeing, while the overweight participants said they exercised to manage their weight. The overweight participants also weighed themselves daily or weekly to see if they had lost weight from all their hard work at the gym, which they still believed wasn't enough. And when that scale didn't move down, they felt bad. Exercising because you want to lose weight rather than because you want to feel good turns something positive into something negative.

If you know my story, you know that I didn't lose weight until I was injured and did absolutely nothing because my body so badly needed rest to heal. If doing nothing feels good, then you absolutely need to do nothing. If doing nothing makes you feel bad, get off your butt and move! Check in with your body, moment to moment, to gauge how you feel and what your body needs. Every moment is different.

The first question you want to ask yourself is, "Why am I really moving?" Is it for fun? To release stress? To increase energy? Increase strength and endurance? If those are your answers, you probably don't have a problem fitting movement into your life. If you're moving for another reason, such as strictly to lose weight or because you think you have to, you're likely dreading it.

For a while, my go-to exercise was the stair stepper. I did it because it burned a lot of calories and it was hard. At the time, I told myself that I loved to challenge myself. *It's so hard*, I thought, *I just want to quit, but I keep pushing through. Yay for me!* The entire time I was on the machine, I was counting down the minutes until I was finished. Afterward, I gave myself a pat on the back because I thought I was going to lose weight.

I completed that exercise day after day for the completely wrong reasons. If I hadn't been concerned about weight loss, I would never have done it. I dreaded it. I did it simply because I thought I was supposed to do it. And yet, it never worked. No matter how much effort I put in, I didn't lose weight on that machine. I have to tell you I haven't stepped on a stair stepper since I had that realization, and I don't miss one minute of it.

It's important to challenge yourself, but there are many ways to do that. I challenge myself with stillness, fearful things, and headstands in yoga. You don't have to challenge yourself by over doing it on a stair stepper; you can challenge yourself in a way that feels good and exciting to you.

Exercise, on its own, has nothing to do with weight loss. I realize that is a challenging statement to believe, however, I cannot find enough consistent correlation between exercise and weight loss to connect the two. Exercise, then, is about feeling good and having fun, and that's what causes weight loss.

Think about those people you know who once were sedentary, then they got a gym membership and suddenly they were excelling–discovering new strengths and hobbies, a whole new community, and a whole new way of being. They felt great, and so their body rewarded them with weight loss. If what you're doing doesn't feel great to you, you'll begin that toxic relationship with the scale.

Challenging yourself with exercise builds strength, both mentally and physically. When you accomplish something you didn't know you could accomplish, like running a mile, and you do it just to prove to yourself that you can, you feel awesome! It's very different than running a mile to lose five pounds. Your body loves to move and release feel-good hormones. It wants to do that, but it only can do it if *you* feel good. That doesn't come from beating yourself up, and your subconscious knows that.

Building strength and endurance, two important components of exercise, also feels good. Therefore, establishing an exercise routine centered on a desire to increase strength or endurance—instead of weight loss—will bring about positive results. If you are consistently exercising, your strength and endurance will increase. It's almost impossible to fail as long as you show up. The same can't be said for weight loss, because there are too many variables involved.

If you're exercising for weight loss, and the scale doesn't go down, it's easy to feel like you've failed, even if you've grown healthier, stronger, or faster. If you exercise for strength or endurance, however, the results are easy to see and feel. After starting a regular routine, you notice you can run without stopping and open the pickle jar. This makes you feel encouraged, instead of discouraged, and your body rewards you for your efforts.

A study was done just last year that compared forced versus voluntary exercise using rats. Instead of benefiting from exercise, the rats that were forced to exercise showed less motivation and higher levels of stress than the rats that exercised voluntarily. The same is true for humans. Our bodies respond with stress when we force ourselves to do things we don't want to do. Therefore, it is imperative that you are experiencing positive emotions while you are exercising. This can only happen if you're engaging in activities you like.

If you aren't sure whether you feel negative, remember that your mind communicates with words and your body communicates with feelings. How does the activity make you *feel*?

It's all about doing something that feels good to you. Be aware of what movements actually release stress and which movements add to your stress. You will be surprised with the results.

Also notice how often you feel like moving. Pay attention to what your body wants and *when* it wants it. We all have heard that it takes a certain number of days to build a habit. However, if exercise is a hobby, something you do for fun, does it need to become a habit? When you love something, you don't have to force yourself to do it or build a habit out of it. It just comes naturally.

In the past we didn't have gyms. We hunted for our food and did chores. That was our exercise. We didn't hop on a treadmill for an hour of exercise while watching TV.

Kids don't think about exercise; they just play. When did we get away from that? Do you ever watch kids run simply to get from point A to point B? Would you ever run to go talk to somebody across the parking lot?

Think about why you do or do not do things. Take showering, for example. Most of us agree that showering is something we want to do most days. It feels good to be clean. We see a direct benefit from doing it, and if we skip it for too long, we crave it strongly. What is the difference between showering, and say, running? Why do you shower effortlessly, yet running takes a pep talk, a large helping of force, and ultimately a "just do it" attitude?

It's about motivation. If running is a passion, something you feel like you were born to do and something you excel at, your attitude will most likely be, "I get to run today!" You'll be excited. If running is something you do because you told yourself you would, it has been shown to aid in weight loss, or because it will let you check off an I-exercised-today box, you will likely feel sluggish and bored.

What if you felt about exercise the same way you feel about showering? What if, when you skipped it for too long, you started to crave it desperately? You can have that reality, but you have to choose exercise that makes you feel good or you won't get those benefits. You also have to choose it for the right reasons. If you choose exercise for weight loss, and you don't lose weight, you will ignore the other benefits it gives you. That's a problem.

I never had an exercise routine until I was trying to lose weight. All of a sudden I *had* to work out at least five days a week. I *had* to work out for a certain amount of time. I had to sweat a certain amount and burn enough calories to feel like I did the job. Coincidentally, this was the period I gained the most weight.

Before I exercised for weight loss, if I felt like moving I did. If I didn't, I wouldn't. I never worried that if I stopped doing something I would never return to it. I knew that if I took a month off it wouldn't be long before I was right back into the swing of things.

Back then, exercising was the same as showering for me. If I didn't exercise, I simply felt different that day. When too many of those days went by, I wanted to do it naturally. Without any force at all. When I disconnected from my body, my relationship with exercise changed.

It all comes back to a basic trust in your body. The body will always take you back to movement; just know that and let it do it for you. You don't have to be an athlete. You don't have to have 15 percent body fat and be able to lift 50 pounds and run five miles. You can just move to move.

Often times, when we search for movement ideas, we compare what we think we might try to outside standards or to other people who are having success. If your friend lost 20 pounds with running, it doesn't mean running will work for you. Your friend might run and completely check out into a place of sheer bliss. You might hate running and feel that it's the most boring activity ever. When you let exercise be the thing that makes you feel stronger, breathe better, overcome limiting beliefs, and create a more balanced body, you'll reap major benefits. When you make it the thing you do only to lose weight or look a certain way, you don't get the same benefits.

I have a friend who once decided she wanted to run with me two times a week. After a few months of running, she told me that she hadn't lost any weight. I hadn't realized we were running so she could lose weight, so I asked her if she liked it. She said she hated running, but she thought if she came out and ran twice a week—when before she was doing nothing—she would lose weight.

Makes sense, right? Most of us would have thought like my friend. If we go from no activity to some activity, then we should lose weight. But my friend didn't take into account how the activity made her feel. She hated running and did it for the wrong reasons. That's when I turned to her and said, "What the heck are we doing this for? I certainly don't like to run, but I do enjoy being a teacher or helping out a friend. But you don't like running so we shouldn't be running!"

The same goes for you. Lifting weights, going to the gym, or running for two months just to lose weight with the intention of stopping afterward will never work. Your body is too smart. So what do you like to do? What can you not live without? What do you look forward to doing the rest of your life?

Turn your movement experience into an opportunity to be grateful. Be grateful you can walk, even if you can't or don't want to run. Be grateful you can choose any movement, and then choose the ones you love.

As with food, being aware with exercise means no distractions allowed. No TV or reading while moving, while you are connecting to your body through awareness. In the future you can multi-task if you want, although I strongly recommend you don't. For now, though, you are in the process of looking for awareness and connection.

Listen to what your body is telling you. What does it want? What feels good? If you are on the bike and you believe the only way you can get through it is to read, then get off the bike for good. Now, if you have a bike at home, and you want to read a magazine but you don't feel like sitting still, then by all means jump on the bike. The important factor is your motivation. Are you on the bike to read a magazine or to get in your movement? Your body can only do one thing at a time efficiently.

If you are having a difficult time connecting with exercise, it's time to get into your soulful hobbies. What makes you happy? Regardless of the level of activity, you have to start somewhere. What is fun for you? What sounds like it might be fun? What have you given up on doing?

Maybe you're an artsy person, and you don't naturally love to move your body seven days a week. If that is what is coming from your soul, and movement isn't on your love-it list, there is nothing wrong with that. Our bodies only want to move when they feel good. They also don't want to move anymore than what feels good, and that amount is different for every person. Get clear about what makes you feel good, and engage in that activity.

Always stick to what you love. If you find you are looking for excuses to skip movement, stop doing movement. You don't need to make excuses. You are allowed to say you don't want to do that movement today. You have the power of free will. If it keeps happening, it's probably time to reconsider your movement choice. It may even be time to take a break from movement altogether, and let your body start to crave it naturally.

Your body is smart. It will never allow you to get through something negative, and then give you positive results. Begin treating your exercise like a hobby, and remove the multi-tasking from it so you can receive the benefits you desire.

Questions for Transformation:

1. **What movements am I currently doing?** Write out all movements, including exercise, chores, and everyday

movements like walking the dog or taking out the trash. Leave nothing out.

2. **How much am I enjoying what I'm doing?** Rate each of the above movements on a scale of 1 to 10, 10 being absolute love.

3. **What movements do I most want to do?** What sounds fun? What do you think would be the movements you would want to do the rest of your life? Nothing more, nothing less.

4. **What movements do I wish I could do?** What movements don't seem feasible at this exact moment in your life but are ones you envision doing in the future?

Once you've answered those questions and brought awareness to your movements, you can begin problem solving. What did you notice about the movements you are currently doing and the ones you would like to be doing? If you remove the goal of weight loss from exercise, does this change how you see it?

If you're finding there are real obstacles (financial or otherwise) in the way of you doing the activities you want to do, then it's time to get creative. If you have the desire to do something, a solution exists. It's just a matter of finding it.

How can you see beyond your limitations and think more creatively? My two-year-old son is learning this skill right now. He sees his chair against the table and decides he wants to sit in it. At first, he tries to sit in it before moving it away from the table. He falls. Then he attempts to pull it out, and it gets stuck. The more he pulls, the more frustrated he becomes. It just keeps getting more stuck. He looks at me crying, begging me to rescue him, and I calmly say, "You can do it, love." This time, he stops pulling. He looks at the chair and the table, and pulls from the bottom of the chair. It easily slides out, and he sits down.

You can go through the same process. Take a deep breath,

step away from the problem, and think creatively. There's always a solution, though it may be different than what you originally thought it would be. If it's something you really want to do, the rewards you'll reap from the movement will definitely make it worth finding a solution.

Live Intentionally

Living requires more than simply breathing. While breathing enables us to survive, surviving isn't the same as living. It's barely living. In fact, the APA released an article stating that a third of Americans are "extremely stressed" and almost half (48 percent) are living in an ever-increasing stress response.

To be alive, we must go beyond that space of survival. We must live with intention.

Living with intention requires us to dig deep and recognize our limiting beliefs, excuses, and lack of clarity. We tend to assume that our goals and motivations are clear. We may ask, "I want to lose weight, what else do I need to know?" There is so much more to the story than simply weighing less. That's like saying, "I want a piece of cake." There are hundreds of different types of cake and if you have your heart set on carrot cake and get chocolate, you may not be happy. Intention allows us to become clear about exactly what we want, why we want it, and what's getting in the way of achieving it.

If you are feeling stuck, this is the step that will help you move forward with intention and direction. The last step allowed you to become aware of where you are beginning.

This step helps you clear the space to choose a path to follow. And not just any path—the exact right path for you for long-term results in your body and life.

Total Body Transformation:

In 1943, Abraham Maslow published a paper on human motivation that outlined a hierarchy of needs. He organized these needs in a five-tiered pyramid where each level depends on the subsequent level below.

The five tiers (from bottom to top):

1. Physiological needs: Food, water, warmth, and rest;

2. Safety needs: Security and safety;

3. Belongingness and love needs: Intimate relationships and friends;

4. Esteem needs: Prestige and feeling of accomplishment;

5. Self-actualization: Achieving one's full potential, including creative activities.

The first two tiers are considered basic needs. In my opinion, if all you want is to lose weight, you simply need to fully satisfy those two basic tiers. If you want more—if you want to transform your life—you need to fulfill those needs and then focus on the others, as well.

The three upper tiers of the pyramid are considered self-fulfillment needs. Fulfilling these needs comes from living with intention. The truth is not all thin people are living with intention. Not all thin people are self-actualized and achieving their full potential, but the ones who are truly living their best lives in their best bodies are.

And so, once again, if your goal here is to simply weigh less, all you have to do is understand your intention, fulfill your basic needs, and expect your body to self correct. Then your work is done.

However, if you choose to live a full and vibrant life, you will want to learn more about this idea of living with intention. You won't be sorry.

Total Life Transformation:

Step One: Acknowledge Excuses

According to Maslow, self-actualized people share similar traits. These traits:

Able to tolerate uncertainty;

Accepting of themselves and others;

Spontaneous;

Problem-centered instead of self-centered;

Creative;

Appreciative and grateful for life at the basic level;

Fully aware;

Comfortable with risk;

Internally driven (meaning they listen to internal voice and feelings instead of external voices);

Responsible; and

Able to acknowledge and work on their weaknesses.

These traits are not to be taken lightly. Most of them cause extreme discomfort at first because they involve the need for change. Change is scary, and fear is where the mind can get stuck. And, when it does, our fear becomes the main contributor to an overall inability to lose or maintain weight.

To move forward, begin to look at how you show up in these other areas of your life. For example, how do you show up with relationships? Are you willing to settle for a relationship that is not ideal for you? Do you have a pattern where you seek out relationships that are unsupportive to confirm your belief that you are not supported? Sometimes we may even tolerate abuse out of a misguided perception that we have done something to deserve it. The same goes for our weight. We may believe that we deserve a body that is not ideal because of our past choices and experiences.

If we are operating from this mindset and we choose our exercises, we may choose punishing exercises in order to beat ourselves up for gaining weight or being out of control. We also may create unrealistic expectations in order to prove that we don't follow through with anything and can't be trusted. Instead of figuring out what motivates us, we may then begin to believe that we are not meant to exercise and even that we don't like to move.

Many people also settle in their careers, allowing themselves to work in jobs that don't meet their needs or are unsatisfying. They will accept low pay when they should be demanding more or work overtime for a boss instead of asking for rest when they need it. The fear of disapproval or security becomes so overwhelming that they convince themselves this is what they have to do. The same goes for their weight. They become so afraid of failure that they choose to do the same things they have done over and over again, even if they don't work long-term.

These mindsets are rooted in fear, and they lead to life circumstances that cause many people to gain weight. Once we figure out what our fears are, however, and how they're manifesting in our lives, it becomes easy to drop the weight. The challenging part is tackling the fear.

It is my experience that the process of weight loss described in this book is not as front loaded as with many other weight-loss programs. In other words, you may be used to starting a program, losing weight, and then hitting a wall. This process doesn't allow any trickery so you may not lose large amounts of weight up front. However, once you push through the fears, the weight comes off, and it stays off.

To get there, though, you must acknowledge and eliminate the excuses your mind uses to keep you stuck. You may feel ready for change. You could very well be amped up and ready to go, but your mind has two very effective tools that get in the way: vividness and availability.

Our minds cling to emotion. They prefer the personal and emotional to something potentially more concrete. This is the trickery of vividness. Advertisers use this often by showing you a commercial that plays on an emotion even if there isn't evidence to back up their claims.

Availability, on the other hand, is a mind trick where we unconsciously decide to accept something because we already have stored information on that subject in the past. If we have prior knowledge of something, regardless if it's true or not, we are more likely to accept the information and ignore conflicting information, even if the conflicting information is backed by scientific evidence.

It is important to understand how these two mind tricks can get in the way of proper critical thinking and evaluation. For example, say you want to go to the gym after work. And let's assume that it's truly a desire of yours, not something you are forcing yourself to do to lose weight. You pack your bag and think about it all day. It feels good in your body, and you know it's going to be positive and uplifting. All of a sudden, around 3:00 p.m., the excuses begin.

Maybe I shouldn't go to the gym, you think. Then the irrational thoughts begin, *I saw on the news this morning that you're not supposed to go the gym consecutive days in a row*, or *Sally said she was getting pizza after work and I like pizza; it makes me feel so comforted and happy*. The first thought utilizes availability by linking information together to create sound evidence in your mind. The second thought uses vividness by connecting an emotion to pizza, which makes it irresistible.

You begin to hear thoughts like these: *I don't have time to go the gym. I'm so tired I should probably relax. My knee will probably flare up*, etc. The mind in crisis mode starts feeding you all these excuses that leave you feeling confused and out of sorts.

The mind in the grip of fear also will try to make you believe you're a victim. You may find yourself thinking, *I was born with this body, I can't change it; All of my family is overweight, it's hereditary;* or *I have tried everything, there is something wrong with me.*

None of these is true. It is my belief that if you have the desire to release your excess weight, you have the ability to succeed. If you have a family history of high cholesterol, high blood pressure, or heart disease, you still have the ability to make choices that help you avoid a similar fate.

Epigenetics has gifted us the power of choice. It states that our genetics are not fixed. That our environment actually influences our ability to turn genes on and off. And so we can feel empowered that our life is not predetermined or destined in any way.

Just as you have a choice to become a lawyer even if your parents were teachers, you have the choice to be in your ideal body, even if your parents struggle with weight. When your mind is programmed to be overweight, which it often is when one or both parents struggle with weight, it is simply a matter of intentionally reprogramming yourself.

A client we will call Sue struggled with emotional eating and weight her entire life. In order to deal with her excess weight, she became addicted to exercise. She ran miles and miles to keep her body thin. She always reached her goal weight temporarily, and then strived to weigh less. After striving to weigh even less, she'd eventually gain the original weight back. She described her mom as having the same tendencies and felt as though her fate would be the same, purely through genetic predisposition.

Over time, we worked together to eliminate her emotional eating behaviors. Before long, she was eating when she was hungry and stopping when she was full. She wasn't feeling deprived, and she wasn't cutting calories anymore. Her exercise was back in balance as something she did purely for enjoyment and not to make up for the calories she ate.

Her body began to respond. She was able to achieve her goal weight and stay there, using this process—a process Sue described as freeing rather than enslaving. She changed her programming and began living as someone who doesn't have a weight problem. She allowed her behaviors to mimic that of a naturally thin person and watched her body easily and effortlessly transform. She now feels confident that her issues with weight and food are forever behind her. You can do the same.

Part of acknowledging and eliminating excuses is recognizing when you're engaging in pitiful thinking. A scared mind may trigger a pity party, and you might find you start thinking thoughts like: *Poor me, I gained all this weight. How could I have let myself get here; I'm so pathetic. I obviously don't care at all about healthy living. I can't believe I've done this to myself. I can't do anything right. I look awful. No one loves me.*

These thoughts aren't helpful. Having gained weight is not the end of the world. Millions of people struggle with weight. It doesn't say anything about you except that you have a skill to learn and develop. If you dwell on how you got to where you are, however, and engage in self-pity, you will stay where you are or continue to gain.

Your past happened. It's done. It's now time to see your potential.

If you feel like you can't tell the difference between excuses and truth, listen to your feelings. In yoga, there is an emphasis on body communication. The belief is that your body sends you messages though symptoms and feelings. Your body is then the mediator between your internal and external worlds, giving you the information you can't always experience directly with your senses.

If you hear your mind say, "You need to rest today," consider how that statement feels in your body. Does it feel relieving? Does it feel guilt ridden? Does it feel like a way to keep you stuck? If the excuse creates a negative emotion, don't listen to it.

If you are sitting on the couch thinking, *I should be at the gym*, bring your attention to your next emotion. Do you feel bad? Negative thoughts may sound like this: *I know that's what I should do Why didn't I go? Why am I sitting here?* Or do you feel good? Positive thoughts may sound like this: *Oh, yeah. That's what I need. Moving would feel so good!*

You may also feel relieved. You may feel your body relaxing and hear yourself thinking, *Oh yes. I feel like resting today. That sounds so good!*

Always follow what makes you feel better. Make a decision and own it. It doesn't even matter if it is the "right" one, as long as you own it. Your body recognizes uncertainty and doesn't like it. Be intentional.

If you choose to work through your workout, own that decision. If you choose to eat out, own that decision. If you can't own it, don't do it. If you can't own eating that food, or going to the gym, don't do it.

If you are feeling lazy, either get up and move or be lazy and proud! If you think all naturally thin people aren't lazy you are mistaken. The difference is that naturally thin people don't have any negative emotions around their levels of activity. My research showed that non-dieters choose movement often, but also do not feel bad if they choose to skip it. They're connected to their bodies, and they make intentional decisions about movement and food.

Acting with intention emphasizes choice, and the experience of having choices enables us to stay empowered. To get the most out of each day, check in with yourself often and ask, "What would I rather be doing?" If your answer is, "Nothing! I'm having a blast!" that's great. If you can come up with an answer that is different than what you are doing, make the choice to do that instead. If you're not happy with what you're doing but you can't come up with an answer for what you'd rather be doing, you may be looking to numb out and not be present. If that is the case, get up right away and go do anything else. Assuming, that is, that your goal is to live a life that is present instead of numb.

It is always easier to stay the same than it is to change. It's easier to give up than to go after what you want. It's easier to be numb than present. It's easier to gain weight than to lose it, if that's what you are used to doing. Just as it's easier to lose weight than gain it for the group of people who complain about being too skinny. Although it may be hard to empathize with this group of people, they are often in as much pain as those who struggle to lose weight and feeling just as insecure about their bodies.

It's uncomfortable to change. It's uncomfortable to push yourself and stand up for yourself. Easy is not the natural approach for a human being, however. We like challenge, growth, and education. As much as we hate change, we also can't get enough of it.

This process of losing weight shouldn't be hard and torturous, but if it's really easy and you aren't growing, learning, and changing, the likelihood of long-term success is slim to none. Tony Robbins describes this as "disciplining your disappointment." He says that if achieving what you desire were easy, then you wouldn't value it. The value and fulfillment come from going after what you want and never giving up. With weight loss, you are working to make huge transformational shifts to live the life of your dreams. This can't happen without growth and change.

Traditional weight-loss methods often are extreme, punishing, and restrictive. This method isn't, and therefore you often will hear me refer to my approach as easy. However, that doesn't mean it isn't challenging. It is, but it should feel good to grow. It's about getting comfortable with it being uncomfortable.

Exercises for Transformation:

1. Write down ALL of your excuses for not living the life you want. Don't hold back. This is the time to step into the fear, the victimhood, the pity party—all of it. Much of what you write will be irrational and illogical. This is normal. Write it anyway. You need to see what's going on in your mind so you can move through it.

2. Each time you notice these excuses, make a conscious choice to acknowledge them as excuses. Then choose your next step. You can choose to numb out. You can choose to eat outside of hunger. You can choose to skip the gym. Just allow it to be a choice.

3. Write out all the desires that you've ever had in your lifetime. Include the desires you had as a child. Don't hold back here. Imagine you had a magic genie or fairy godmother who could give you everything you want, no questions asked. Allow yourself to write everything you could ever want without limiting yourself.

4. Look at your list, and see if you can begin grouping your desires together. For example, maybe you desire to be a size six and you desire to exercise more. Those desires could go together. Once you finish grouping things together, look at each grouping and ask yourself, "What's the common underlying desire here?" For example, maybe you desire to be a size six and exercise more because you assume this would

bring you greater health. The underlying desire, then, is health or peace from the fear of sickness. Discover the underlying desires that you have attached to these external events, and then ask yourself, "How else might I achieve more of this desire?" How can you find more peace besides being a size six? How can you feel healthier besides exercising more? How can you find more peace and health in this moment as opposed to attaching it to a future external event?

Step Two: Identify Limiting Beliefs

In the movie *Facing the Giants*, a football player states his reservations about playing a team that he perceives is better than his. The coach asks him to get on the ground and do the death crawl, which requires him to use his hands and feet (knees off the ground) to move across the football field with another player on his back. The coach then states that the player will be doing it blindfolded so that he can't see how far he's gone. The coach knows that the football player has a perception of how many yards he can go, and he wants to remove this barrier. And so, with his limitations lifted, the player death crawls the entire football field with a man on his back.

We all have these limits in our minds. They keep us stuck and safe, and it becomes easier to believe them than to change them. These limiting thoughts are extremely powerful and feel valid and true, but they're not.

Recently, I put a client on the chest fly machine where he proceeded to do 15 repetitions just like I asked. He then looked down and expressed his surprise at the weight. He thought the weight was set at 62.5 pounds. I had moved it to 75 pounds without his knowledge. He admitted that had he known it was at 75 pounds, he would have assumed he could only do a few repetitions at best.

That assumption would have been wrong.

Many of us hold the same type of incorrect assumptions about our weight. A study conducted on hotel maids several years ago showed this same truth. The hotel maids were highly active all day, yet the majority of them were overweight. The researchers asked the maids if they exercised regularly. The maids all claimed that they did not. The researchers found this interesting since they were clearly active all day long as they cleaned rooms, pushed heavy carts around, and did laundry.

The researchers decided to split the maids into two groups. The first group served as the control group. The researchers then showed the maids in the second group how active they really were. They showed the maids an average calorie burn per day and how they far exceeded the minimum daily exercise requirement.

After just one month, that group of maids lost weight. Without changing anything but their perception.

The mind uses confirmation bias to give weight to any evidence that is congruent with our current beliefs, while ignoring threatening information. And because our beliefs have years of experience to back them up, it becomes difficult to change them. Difficult, however, is not impossible.

Logic and reasoning are developed somewhere around the age of five in most children. Prior to this development, we are highly susceptible to the information around us. This is mostly to our advantage so that we can learn quickly. Our sponge-like brains are able to quickly absorb what's happening around us so we can develop at a rapid pace. The disadvantage, however, is that we are not selective in what we take in.

What we experienced as children shapes our adult lives. If you believe you aren't worth much as a child, you could grow up with self-worth issues. If you believe you aren't safe, then you could have issues with security and safety. If you believe life is hard, then it will most likely fulfill that prophecy.

The only way to change this is to change the belief. As soon as you can identify your limiting beliefs, you can change them. But if you ignore them, they will create patterns and habits you carry with you for life.

The good news is beliefs can change in an instant. The speed of a belief change is completely dependent on your willingness to change it. The more open-minded and flexible you are the quicker you will change your beliefs. Some people have made the necessary shifts in a couple of hours. For others, the process takes longer. Your journey is to notice how you limit yourself, and then seek to disprove these limitations.

This isn't easy. Our minds are constantly searching for congruency. When an alternate threatening belief is introduced, the average person will reject it rather quickly in order to avoid cognitive dissonance. Then, to make matters worse, the mind will search for a belief that supports the current belief in order to soften any remaining discomfort from the new idea. And so most people walk around rarely changing their core belief systems.

Therefore, it takes a conscious effort to change. Ask yourself, "How long do I want to continue to put up with these beliefs that aren't serving me?" You get to choose what you believe. Even if you have all the evidence in the world to believe something, you still always have choice. Nothing is fixed or predetermined for you.

Take these two beliefs for example: *Some people are naturally thin, but I am not*; and *I have not yet learned the skillset necessary to live naturally thin*. Which feels better?

The first belief takes away your power to change. It renders some people lucky, and you unlucky. It sets up a life of struggle, as your desire to live without fear of weight gain will be in conflict with your belief that you can't actually achieve that.

The second belief is an accurate description of what is happening right now in your life. Your parents, society, and culture taught you many skills, but living naturally thin simply wasn't one of them. Yet.

Thankfully, you can learn the skillset and have what you desire. Just as you can teach me how to do something that I don't know how to do at this moment, I can teach you how to live naturally thin. First, though, you must commit to changing your beliefs.

You most likely have many beliefs about weight, food, and exercise that are not in service to your desires. You may desire freedom around food, and yet your belief tells you that food makes you fat. Or perhaps you don't trust yourself when given freedom with food, and so you hold on with tight control regardless of what you desire. You may want to crave exercise, but you believe that you *have* to exercise because you ate food. Therefore, your desires and your beliefs are in conflict with one another. These conflicts will keep you stuck.

Even once you realize this conflict, you may find yourself fighting desperately to keep your old beliefs. Remember: The mind is very good at this.

People will often argue with me about how weight loss works in order to subconsciously defend their belief systems, even though those beliefs are not the ones they want. It becomes too painful to admit their current beliefs are potentially inaccurate. They tell me that nobody can truly be thin without dieting, and I am a fraud for teaching otherwise. And yet they struggle every day to live in their ideal body using traditional dieting methods.

It is easier to believe the traditional dieting methods because it's what the mind is comfortable with. It is information that has been reinforced for years. It's uncomfortable to adopt a new belief system that causes conflict in the mind—even if it actually feels better to think in this other way.

Commit to changing anyway.

Take a look at your limiting beliefs about weight. What beliefs can you acknowledge, in this moment, that are in conflict with what you desire? You can trust your desires over your limiting beliefs.

Also pay attention to other beliefs that may influence your weight loss journey. For example, do you have a drive for perfection? Are you seeking the perfect diet, perfect amount of exercise, and the perfect body? The false sense of perfection will limit your ability to transform into the unique person that you are. Nobody is perfect. However, magazines and television give an impression of perfection through lighting, make up, and digital touch up. Human beings in the real world, however, have imperfections.

Begin to look beyond the weight. If your body keeps giving you weight to tell you to change something and the change that needs to be made is to increase your self-love, can you imagine what it would be like to learn to love yourself no matter what size and shape you are? What an amazing lesson to be learned!

Some of you gain weight due to life circumstances, like a toxic work environment or low-quality relationship. So although you may make small changes to release weight temporarily, your body is asking more of you to live in your best body and life. If this is you, your weight can become your most incredible motivator to have everything you desire, far beyond a smaller body.

For some of you, weight is acting as protection or a way to hide. With excess weight, you perceive you can hang out in the background and nobody will notice you. If you were to step out and into the light you may have to deal with attention, judgment, criticism, or any other outside percep-tions you don't want. If that is your reality, a smaller body might simply make you feel more vulnerable. In that case, it would be imperative to notice such beliefs around needing to hide, and choose instead to be seen, no matter how un-comfortable that is at first.

Exercises for Transformation:

Write down ALL of your limiting beliefs around weight, food, exercise, and your body. Pay attention to your beliefs surrounding your ability to succeed. Do you really think it's possible to live in your ideal body? Do you feel stuck in the fate of your parents? Just as you can choose any career you desire regardless of your parents, you can choose a differ-ent amount of weight.

Step Three: Find Clarity

What do you really want from weight loss? What is the final result or the end goal?

We tend to think in the terms of when I lose weight ... then I will have. You may think, *If I was smaller I would feel more at-tractive, then I would find love.* But a smaller body is no guar-antee you will meet Prince Charming or the love of your life, just like a larger one is not a guarantee you won't.

Losing weight is never a guarantee that anything will come true. The truth is the only thing weight loss guarantees is that you weigh less. Any other meaning beyond that is unre-liable. In fact, if you force your body to get smaller without taking into consideration the internal shifts necessary for long-term change, you often will not experience any of the results you thought you would.

This is why it's imperative that you shift into the person you want to become now.

Pay attention to the journey you are choosing to release ex-cess weight. If you lose weight in a manner that isn't loving and accepting or that doesn't give you confidence, then it will be virtually impossible to achieve these things once you lose the weight.

The good news is that you can have all the feelings you desire deeply from weight loss *at this time.* You don't have to wait until the scale reads the number you desire so deeply. The scale will only tell you what you weigh. It will never tell you who you are or how to feel. You choose a feeling based on past programing and limiting beliefs.

Work to discover what your motivating factors are for losing weight. Do you want more money? To live longer? To look better in clothes? To get a better job? What have you attached to weight loss? Write out what you want to gain from losing weight, and then get honest with yourself that weight loss is not a guarantee of these things. Learn to recognize that if you're not experiencing these things now, a smaller body is not the correct path to achieve them.

These false expectations given to weight are dysfunctional. It leads you to a path of weight loss full of impatience, urgency, and a large degree of defeat when the scale begins moving down but your personal circumstances don't change.

At first you will feel excited about your weight loss, but just as moving to another state to escape your problems doesn't work, moving to a new body to feel differently won't either. Your job is to get to the root of why you are not experiencing your dream life today, regardless of what is happening externally.

I heard a story from Wayne Dyer that explains this perfectly. Let's say the power went out in your home just as you were getting ready to leave. At this point, it's pitch black, and you want nothing more than to find your keys. You frantically feel around in the dark for your keys, but without light, it's a major struggle.

You notice the streetlights are on so you walk outside into the street. You begin looking around on the street for your keys, and your neighbor walks out.

"What are you looking for?" he asks.

"My keys," you reply. "I dropped them."

He begins to look around and then finally asks, "Where did you drop them?"

"In the house," you reply, "but I thought I'd go out to where the light was to find them."

We all see the absurdity of that story. Why on earth would you walk outside to search for something you were looking for inside? If the keys are located in the house, you can find them only inside of the house. And yet so many of us live that absurdity on a regular basis. Everything we truly desire—more confidence, happiness, health, love, etc.—is located on the inside, yet we too often search outside to receive them.

Intentional living requires clarity about what you truly want and where you can find it. You must stop looking for your keys out in the street and learn to turn the light on in the house. If the power is out, find a flashlight. Light up the true answers within you so that you can actually find what you are seeking. The questions below can help.

Questions for Transformation:

1. **What are my top 20 strengths?** We all have unique talents and strengths that have shaped who we are. Get in touch with what those are. Write them down.

2. **What do I really want beyond a smaller or more toned body?** What do you desire deeply on the inside that you have attached to weight loss? Write down these things. How can you begin creating these in your current reality?

3. **What's getting in my way?** What obstacles are currently getting in the way of you achieving your ideal body and life? What lies are you telling yourself that are holding you back that you are now realizing aren't true at all?

Live Joyously

Living from a place of joy is the most important gift we can give ourselves, and we can use weight as a motivation to achieve this blissful state. Joy often becomes blocked by excess stress and lack of gratitude. When stress takes over our lives, it becomes challenging to think positively and feel good. Stress also has a profound effect on the body. This step focuses on understanding those effects and finding strategies to move out of a place of stress and into a place of gratitude where joy can be experienced.

Total Body Transformation:

If all you want is to be thin, you don't have to live joyously. Thin people, even naturally thin people, experience stress, and there are many who lack gratitude and joy. If you simply want to weigh less, all you have to do in this step is give your body the tools it needs to burn fat efficiently.

In other words, you need to trick your body into believing it's relaxed long enough for it to step out of fight or flight mode and into fat burning mode.

When the body is under stress, or living in survival mode, it has no need to efficiently burn fat. In fact, it would prefer to *store* fat, as that aids its efforts to survive danger. Most people, then, will at least temporarily gain weight in a stressful environment, though that is not true for everyone. If the person has an underlying belief that they can't or don't gain weight, this belief can override the body's natural tendency to pack on the pounds under stress.

Being that you most likely don't have such a belief yet, your job—if you want to be thin—is to give your body every available tool so that it can burn fact more optimally. Eventually, you will move into beliefs about your body that are better equipped to deal with stress, but until then these tools can help:

1. Breathe deeply and often. Set a timer to remind you to take five to 10 deep breaths every hour (or whatever time period feels appropriate to you). Breathing deeply shifts the body from stress to relaxation. The more often you do this, the better chance your body has to burn fat.

2. Meditate. Spending a significant amount of time in a relaxed state, as one does meditating, can help the body easily burn fat. I like to use guided meditations, which are available online for free (MeditationOasis.com). Or you can choose from multiple apps on your phone or tablet.

3. Practice restorative yoga. Schedule a restorative yoga class into your calendar each week to help balance the busyness of everyday life. These classes are designed to shift your body out of fight-or-flight and into relaxation.

4. Take a relaxing vacation. I know in the past vacation time may have been a time you gained weight, not lost it. However, a relaxing vacation is the perfect environment for weight loss, assuming you have mastered step one, living connected. Feeling good, having fun, and not worrying about life are all perfect for weight loss.

5. Plan a staycation. Create time in your home that is completely focused on relaxing. If binge watching your favorite TV series is relaxing, not numbing, do it. If lying on your hammock reading sounds blissful, try that. If being active without having to worry about fitting it around your busy schedule sounds appealing, that is great, too. Plan your ideal relaxation time, and let your body rest.

I realize that our society has made relaxing synonymous with laziness, but I have to ask you, how well is going a million miles a minute working for your weight-loss goals? Most likely, your increased stress has not been helping you lose weight, at least not in a healthy, sustainable way. If your body is eating itself for survival, causing you to weigh less, we are not counting that as healthy weight loss.

In order to understand this better, we need to understand the role the nervous system plays in the body. The autonomic nervous system is divided into two parts: the sympathetic and the parasympathetic.

The sympathetic nervous system is responsible for the body's response during a perceived threat. The body responds to this perceived threat by speeding up the heart rate, increasing contractions of the cardiovascular system, and becoming more alert. It triggers the fight-or-flight response, decreases stomach movement and secretions, releases adrenaline, and converts glycogen to glucose for muscle energy.

The parasympathetic nervous system is responsible for the body at rest. The body responds to rest by returning to a state of calm, decreasing heart rate, relaxing the muscles, increasing stomach movement and secretions, and turning off any involvement of the adrenals and the glycogen-to-glucose conversion. It triggers rest and digestion, and it is the state in which our body is meant to spend the majority of its time.

The fight-or-flight response is meant to be a response we use only in case of a threat, yet most people are spending the majority, it not all, of their time there. This causes a major problem with weight and metabolism because digestion *only* happens in relaxation. So take some deep breaths, relax, and allow your body to start burning fat. That's what it is designed to do!

Total Life Transformation:

If you would like to experience a profound sense of relaxation and joy, you'll need to dive deeper into coping with stress and living in gratitude. If you can learn to do that, you'll truly be living your best life.

Step One: Handle Stress

As mentioned previously, stress forces the body into a state of survival. In this survival state, the body will naturally store more fat. This system handles life-or-death scenarios efficiently and effectively, but it isn't such a great system for the everyday, when so many people are living with chronic stress. It's particularly problematic for those trying to lose weight.

Specifically, those of you who struggle with weight likely will have excess stress about excess weight. This means that every time you walk by a mirror, you're likely experiencing more stress, which causes your body to retain ever-greater amounts of fat. This isn't helpful! Thankfully, it can be changed.

Change isn't easy, though. I would love nothing more than to write a sentence that allows you to never feel stressed about your body ever again, but alas, that isn't how it works. So the very first step to transformation is to remove the word stress from your vocabulary.

When you force yourself to think beyond the word stress, you will have to become more accurate in your descriptions of your experiences. For example, when feeling what you previously described as stress, you will have to choose a word that is more accurate. Common words are overwhelmed, exhausted, depressed, anxious, etc.

This may appear to be nothing more than word play, but

remember, your body takes direct orders from your mind. So if you think, *I am stressed*, the body responds with the spike in cortisol and the fight-or-flight state you have become too familiar with. If you choose another word, your body will have to pause to choose its reaction. If you're feeling overwhelmed, for instance, your body may not have an automatic response. Instead, your mind will have to jump in and problem solve from an accurate place, perhaps by removing something from your plate, saying "no" to a request, or simply asking for help.

Stress also seems to lessen when we are making progress toward our desires. We become obsessed with what we don't like when we feel helpless or hopeless in achieving what we want. Therefore, the simple act of reading this book, and feeling like you are in control of your destiny and moving closer to your desires, should relieve a lot of your uneasiness. So allow this process to be your stress reliever and make it a priority to relax as much as possible—especially at mealtimes.

Remember: Digestion happens in a relaxation state. It's why those embarrassing gurgles are so loud when we're in yoga or getting a massage. When the body is under stress, it cannot perform the basic tasks of eliminating what it doesn't need and holding on to what it does. This directly influences metabolism.

It is assumed that people who are naturally thin have faster metabolism. This isn't necessarily true. Instead, although they too may be eating under stress, they have that magical belief that they will remain thin no matter what. This belief overrides the body's need to store fat. Therefore, they don't have to pay attention and relax as much as you do. In the future, you also will have this belief. For now, though, it is crucial to support your body's natural responses and make relaxing during mealtimes a priority.

Next, let's look at how you cope with stress. Do you have

coping strategies, or do you rely on whatever reaction comes up at the time of stress? Stressors will always be part of life. Our job is to do our best to fill ourselves up in order to cope better when those inevitable stressors arrive.

I have never felt the physical effects of stress more than when I had a newborn in my home and was exhausted from sleep deprivation. I had no coping strategies available with such low reserves and found myself feeling completely insane most days. Whether or not you, too, have a newborn in your home, low reserves are a problem when dealing with stressors.

Sleep is a crucial piece of building your coping strategies. Without proper rest, you will find it difficult to deal with even the smallest stressors. If sleep is an issue for you, I highly recommend getting the help you need. Ask your doctor for ideas on where to start.

Proper hydration and high-quality food also help you cope with stressors. We all know how unpleasant we can be if we become too hungry. Utilizing basic self-care techniques will be your best chance at building up your reserves to deal with stressors. Keep high-quality snacks on hand and ensure you have constant access to clean water. Then find those things that make you smile no matter what: a *Friends* episode, a cup of tea, a hot bubble bath, a song, a phone call with a friend, a hug from your significant other, or whatever fills you with joy.

Creative exercises also promote relaxation. Personally, I love coloring, and I engage in it often, doing so even before I knew it was a proven stress reliever. When I focus on coloring, I fall into a child-like state, intent on nothing but staying in the lines. There have been many times that I have stopped in the middle of my work day and colored to relive stress. It's relaxing and fun!

Reducing the negative dialogue in your mind is also a powerful way to cope with stress. The best strategy to do this is to master the process of trust. Trust in yourself, and trust in some spiritual higher power.

Call it whatever you want but trust that you are not alone, that there is a higher power happy to deliver a life you desire once you tap into it. Without trust in something higher than you, the process of life can be a struggle because you're forced to do it alone. It's very difficult to achieve your desires alone.

Whatever higher power or universal law you decide to trust, however, you can be assured that this higher power believes that you don't have to struggle, that you can go through life with ease. We are made of 70 percent water, after all; we are meant to flow through life! Start flowing by embracing spirituality.

In those times when you feel like there is no solution or no way out, you can turn to this higher power or source for help instead of stressing. When I don't know how to solve a problem, I close my eyes, breathe, and thank the universe for sending me the answers I am seeking. I can feel the difference in tension immediately. Faith is a powerful stress reducer!

Remember: Stress does play a role in life so it's not as if you are seeking to remove any and all stress. This is about eliminating unnecessary stress that causes you pain and moves you further from your desires. If you have been trying to lose weight for any amount of time, you're under stress, and it's crucial you begin to release this before your body can truly release pounds permanently. Your job is to seek relaxation as much as possible in order to balance out your system.

Questions for Transformation:

1. **How strong are my current reserves?** Are you in a position to handle stressors effectively? If you have low reserves, it's time to come up with a plan to fill them. Giving yourself

what you need is crucial for your ideal body and life.

2. **What sort of eater am I?** If you are thinking about how many calories you are eating and how you should eat less, you are stressing your body. If you are eating fast and worrying about paying bills, you are stressed. Use deep breathing to transition your mealtimes into relaxing experiences where your body can digest and metabolize optimally.

3. **What sort of exerciser am I?** Although exercise is meant to help reduce stress, some of you will feel adverse effects from exercise if it's too intense for your already stressed body. Check in with your body to make sure that the movements you are choosing are best supporting your body for where it is today. If you are majorly stressed, a spin class may not be the best choice. For some of you will be perfect, but if you are craving gentle yoga it's a good sign you need a slower type of movement instead.

4. **What are my external stressors?** Which ones are constant? Which ones can you eliminate? Begin to put together a plan to reduce these outside stressors as much as possible.

5. **What are my internal stressors?** How are your thoughts or actions contributing to your stress levels? Begin to recognize how you add unnecessary stress to your life and work to eliminate this behavior.

6. **What are my coping strategies?** Brainstorm ways to deal with stressors when they inevitably arise. Think of ways in which you can easily shift out of reactive mode and into a space where you can make clear decisions.

Step Two: Practice Gratitude

When you begin to shift the way you see things, the things you see change. Suddenly, you feel lighter and less burdened. Instead of thinking you need to book a vacation to feel joy, you experience absolute joy just eating dinner with your family.

To truly transform your life, learn to find the joy in ordinary moments. A study was done that asked grieving individuals what they missed most about their loved ones. They all expressed ordinary moments. The way their loved ones mispronounced "pellow" for "pillow," or the way they used to send silly text messages that were so challenging to decode. They all said they missed the hugs and the sound of their loved ones' voices.

We think we need extravagant events to feel joy, yet joy lives within the most ordinary of things. As I look at my son, I do my best to find the joy in the simplest of things because I know I will miss them most when he is grown. Washing his hair at bath time, hearing the way he pronounces the dog's name, laughing uncontrollably during peek-a-boo.

Living in a place of gratitude is shifting into the present and accepting what is happening around us. Please do not confuse gratitude with never-ending positivity. It is imperative to a full-life experience that we feel a full range of emotions, even the unpleasant ones. Gratitude on a hard day may be as simple as stating gratitude in our ability to feel.

Some days, we may need to scream or cry with no gratitude whatsoever. It's important, however, that before long we are able to transition back into a state of honesty and gratitude, that we acknowledge the struggle in our day, and then express gratitude that we have a bed and shoes.

When you're feeling down, focus on the fact that you have a body that moves, a close friend nearby, or a shirt on your body. Whip out some old birthday cards and read what your loved ones said about you. Or unpack the macaroni art from your daughter's elementary days and reflect on the beauty that lies in children.

Practicing gratitude also increases energy. Energy is one of those unique things in that the less you use it, the less you have of it. If you have drops of energy at 3:00 p.m., for example, it is likely you need to be more energetic, not less. Our energy often dips, however, when we're feeling uninspired or focusing on the negative in our lives. Practicing gratitude can give us plenty of reasons to feel excited about life. With excitement, come fun, passion, and inspiration.

So at 3:00 p.m., how about a comedy break? Or a nature walk? Or a movement break? Find something that makes you feel good and floods you with feelings of gratitude for the world around you.

If you're struggling with this because of negative feelings around your weight, remember that while weighing less would feel good, you can still feel really incredible right now. You are doing the work it takes to achieve your desires. That's something to celebrate! It takes time to master a new skill like living naturally thin. Grant yourself the opportunity to feel good while you practice.

The best part is that with joy, come results. It simply does not work the other way around. Shifting your perspective changes your life. And once you reach a state of happiness, the weight loss it is just an added bonus. It's icing on the cake! Yummmm!

Exercises for Transformation:

1. Take pictures of all the ordinary moments that bring you joy in the present. Make a collage of these pictures and really feel the joy from these seemingly boring things. Think about what you will miss as time passes or if you couldn't do these things or see these people. Fill your body with feelings of joy for all the things and people you already have in your life.

2. Allow yourself to feel a range of emotions. It's okay to have a day where you feel less grateful. If you find you get stuck in that place too long, create a gratitude journal that you can turn to in order to move out of that state. Find

things you can be grateful for most days that are already here.

3. Have fun. Find ways to include more joy, fun, and passion in your life. Make a list of 100 things you want to do that you have made excuses not to do. When you're feeling down or ungrateful, try one and see how much better you feel!

Live Truthfully

In order to live in your ideal body and life you must begin living from a place of truth and honesty. This is where the naturally thin have an advantage. They understand that their body is thin. They believe this to their very core. You believe something else entirely. Perhaps that you were genetically predisposed for excess fat or that your appetite is too big. You may believe you are un-athletic or lazy. All of these beliefs group into the overall belief that you are not naturally thin and that you are not meant to be naturally thin. This inaccurate thought is the reason for your never-ending weight battle.

Total Body Transformation:

If you want to focus purely on transforming your body, then this step requires you to remind yourself daily that you are actually thin. Yes, I know, it's covered up by excess fat in this moment, but underneath you are thin. Every person on the planet is. So, in order to be thin, you must connect with this part of you. When you begin to think thoughts of heaviness, remind yourself that your ideal body is already there. It's just underneath the heaviness. It's nothing you have to attain or get. It's already inside of you, and the faster you connect with it the faster you will have it.

Attempting to change these thoughts can feel challenging. It is imperative that you keep your emotions out of this step. Your emotions will want to creep in and convince you that you are a heavy person, not a light one. They will remind you of all the years of evidence and the family members modeling it. Your job is to get focused on what is true.

You cannot prove with certainty that you are destined for heaviness. If you had to write a research paper, proving you could not live like the naturally thin, you would find a paper with many claims and very little conclusive evidence. The truth is you don't really know what your body can do. You only know what it has done. Stick with what you can actually say is true.

Your goal here is to keep it simple. Keep the mind focused on what is true. My belief is every person on the planet can have his ideal body if he desires it. But not all do. Keep thinking light thoughts, and allow the mind to mimic that of someone who is already in her ideal body.

If you would like to do more than transform your body, and actually love and appreciate the person looking back at you in the mirror each day, you will want to do more.

Total Life Transformation:

When we live in true acceptance, we are living the most authentic version of our lives. In other words, we are finally being honest with ourselves. We stop beating ourselves up for the past, and we stop obsessing over the future. We become truthful in this exact moment.

This authenticity can happen when someone has a near death experience or a loved one passes. Such gravity brings a level of honesty to the moment. People begin to realize they don't want a tombstone that reads, "She was thin." They want more. Living truthfully means acknowledging and accepting that "more."

Once we get honest about where we are and where we want to be, and we accept both, we have to take an honest assessment of how we are spending our present time. Instead of wasting time thinking about how we spent our time in the past, or dreaming about how we will spend our time in the future, we have to take a truthful look at the current hours we have in front of us.

This level of acceptance and honesty enables our body to relax and focus on the tasks that are most important. It takes the stress off the body to constantly worry about what it has done or what it needs to do. It allows this moment right here to be enough. And that changes everything.

Step One: Practice Self-Acceptance

When discussing acceptance, we must first discuss body image. Accepting our body image means we can look in the mirror and feel positive about what we see, even if we want to change it. This acceptance is one of the differences between the people who are simply thin and those who actually live in a body they are comfortable with. Our goal is to be in the latter group. We will talk more about this later, but first we are going to cover what a negative body image does so we can shift toward a healthy image immediately.

A negative body image is one that causes pain and suffering. In other words, just living in your body each day is a painful experience that drives you to obsessively move toward changing the body. Expert Marc David has found that it also causes: imbalanced dieting, macronutrient imbalances, binge eating, digestive upset, and food deprivation. Mindfulness becomes a nearly impossible state to attain, because the present is far too full of suffering to actually sit in for a while. Whatever you desire to feel—happiness, confidence, radiance, freedom—becomes impossible until the body physically changes to match whatever picture you hold in your mind as "okay." There is no peace in the here and now. And so you are forced to constantly focus on the future, where today's reality is no more.

In my research, the majority of the overweight participants did not like their bodies, while the majority of ideal-weight candidates did. This may not seem shocking, however, the ideal-weight participants didn't describe their bodies as prettier or smaller. They described their bodies as functioning for them. They did not state their easement with their body to be about fitting into clothes or looking a certain way. Their concerns were with how their bodies felt and served them, and their appreciation for that.

The ideal-weight participants trusted their bodies to work for them. In turn, they cared for their bodies in the best way they could. They chose healthy foods and exercised based on health.

The overweight participants, on the other hand, stated less trust in the body and less effort to take care of those bodies. It bears the question, if the desire is to feel better, doesn't it make sense to feel as good as possible in the current body, as opposed to waiting for the ideal body to show up to take care of it?

The overweight participant's negative body image directly contributed to a neglect of the body. This is obviously problematic in the present moment, but it is also an issue for the future. The perception is that when the body changes physically, the body image also will shift from negative to positive. It places weight loss as the link between healthy and unhealthy body image.

The truth is healthy body image comes from healing your relationship with your body, not from changing it physically. In fact, most people who succeed at losing weight still feel anything but thinner, even at their smaller size. This is due to the unhealed disconnection between the body and mind.

Our first task, then, is to heal our body image before the body ever changes physically. This enables the weight-loss process to happen organically, and it allows our physical transformations to stick, as the body and mind are finally connected and in sync.

According to Marc David, a healthy body image is, "Accepting and rejoicing in the body as it is." You'll notice this definition doesn't say that you have to love the way the body looks in this moment. Your healthy body image could be more like, "This doesn't appear to be my ideal body, but it's my body in this moment so I will make the best of it!"

A dear friend of mine explained it this way: If you wanted to buy a brand new car, but needed to save up some money first, you would continue to drive your current car, taking care of it the best way you could. You may be excited about the new opportunity, but wanting a new car doesn't mean that you abandon your current car, or worse, take a bat to it and start making dents. You simply make the best of what you have, and continue moving toward what you desire.

The easiest way to heal your body image is to become embodied, to get back in your body. For our bodies, this may be as simple as looking in the mirror and saying, "I am okay." Instead of avoiding, demeaning, or ignoring it, just become present with it.

Ask it what it needs and begin a consistent dialogue. Write a letter apologizing for abandoning it, and ask for a fresh start. Begin to treat the body the way you would a best friend that you truly love and just had a falling out with. Make your body your priority and trust me, it will reward you.

Notice what your body does do for you as opposed to what it doesn't. Find gratitude and appreciation for the millions of tasks it completes on a daily basis just to keep you alive. Have compassion and empathy for all the challenges it has had to endure, especially any dieting-related task.

Remember: Dieting causes a disconnection between mind

and body, because it asks you to override the body with the intellect. And your body has sat back and allowed this to happen. It may even have attempted to give you what you want, weight loss in the short-term, in spite of your disregard for what it wants and needs. But it didn't work, because you weren't treating your body in the manner it deserves. Your body is truly your best ally. Now is the time to step back into it and work together.

Even if this is the 427th time you have attempted to lose weight, it has no bearing on your success this time around. This time you are different; you are in a different place with a different direction. All those other times you were using the wrong strategy, and so it was never meant to work.

However, even this new strategy won't work if you don't address a negative or unhealthy body image. One sneaky way body image can be unhealthy is via perfectionism.

My clients tend to fall into two camps: the clients who have a significant amount of weight to lose, and would just be happy to weigh what they weighed the first time they started trying to lose weight, and the people who have a smaller amount of weight to lose and are more focused on having "sleek arms" or "a flat tummy." In the case of the second type of client, I keep a listen out for perfection-focused goals that belie an unhealthy body image.

It is hard to resist the images we see in magazines and on television. Even though we know, logically, that these images are not real, and are intensely photoshopped, our minds become fixated on the perfection of them. Our minds like symmetry and these perfect images we see, and without realizing it, we become focused on attaining this "perfect body," which lacks rolls, wrinkles, and dimples.

For your transformation to be permanent, it is imperative that the motivating factor for having a particular kind of body is not a perfection mechanism. In other words, wanting a certain body so that you can be perfect or flawless creates a negative body image, whereas desiring your ideal body, and being open to what that is, creates a healthier and easily manageable body. You cannot sustain your ideal body using a negative body image.

In the past, I was focused on attaining a six-pack under the assumption that personal trainers should have them. In my mind, I linked this physical attribute to the identity of the person I so desperately wanted to be. At the time, I was a new trainer, I had a history of un-athleticism, and I desperately wanted to fit in with my muscular coworkers. The desire for a six-pack didn't come from an honest, true desire of mine—it came from lack of acceptance in myself. And so I began to struggle trying to attain it.

Some of you may find yourself seeking perfection as more of a need for control. Sometimes we feel that as long as we control everything else (weight, looks, exercise, body) then we will be okay. This is where many eating disorders stem from, and why it is imperative that you notice this behavior now. You can find out if this is true for you by asking the following questions: What do you want to control? Is it the unknown? What fears are motivating this perfection obsession? Are you uncomfortable not knowing if you will be okay, safe, loved? If you find that you are struggling with the need to control, this may be an important topic to discuss with a therapist or other trained professional.

Controlling your arms or your tummy or your weight will not control your life. It will not grant you perfection. If you are living under a negative body image, your mind believes the lie that all you have to do is get the "right" body and you will be happy and complete. But, focusing only on getting the arms or stomach you want, and ignoring the true things that need to be changed to make you happier, won't make all of your dreams come true. Instead, focus on finding those other things in life that bring you purpose and drive. Then maybe those arms will come as a bonus.

On our journey to acceptance, we often have to face some major fears. One of the most common fears in acceptance is the idea of passive resignation. Many of us feel that if we accept, we settle.

In the past, you may have given up on losing weight out of desperation, and found yourself heavier than you were before. If that was the case, you may have linked giving up and acceptance as one in the same. In your mind, giving up is the same as throwing up your arms and saying, "I guess it's just not meant to happen for me so I will just be fat and happy." Yet, the happy never seemed to show up, and so you were left with just the fat.

But giving up out of frustration isn't acceptance. Acceptance is different. It says, "Instead of fighting with what is, why don't I make the best of it and also move toward my desire at the same time?" Instead of focusing purely on the destination—a different body—it asks you to focus on where you're starting, as well as the journey it takes to get to your destination.

Let's say there are two people traveling to Paris from California. The first person realized that this long flight might bring about some discomfort, so they booked a first-class ticket, wore the comfiest clothes for the flight, and brought along their most beloved person to chat and watch movies with. They figured if they were going to be on the ride to Paris, they might as well make it as enjoyable as possible.

The second person grumbled and groaned about how long the flight was going to be and how much it was going to cost. So they bought the cheapest ticket they could find on a crappy airline, grabbed whatever clothes were clean (which happened to be uncomfortable), and brought along the most obnoxious person they knew because that person agreed to pay for some expenses upon arrival.

Both people are traveling to the same destination, yet their journeys will be very different. The first traveler has accepted her current location and her journey, and she can't wait to reach her destination so she made the best of it. The second traveler wanted to get to Paris, but was annoyed that the journey was long and expensive and found no enjoyment until the long flight was over.

So here's the question: If I waved my magic wand and made it so that you could not lose or gain another pound, and would therefore have this exact body you're in for the rest of your life, no matter what you did or didn't do, what would you do? Most people would agree that they would make the best of it. They would simply create the best life they possibly could with the body they have. If there is no way to change it, there's really no other choice but to move on and live your life.

The second question is, would you be relived or terrified? For some of you, this thought is terrifying. The idea that you could never have the body you picture in your mind is scary. For most of you, it's relieving. The idea that you don't have to fight this fight anymore is freeing. The reason why it's freeing is because it's true acceptance.

The beauty is that I don't have a magic wand that makes it impossible to lose weight. You get to live from that same place of freedom making the best of the body you have today, while simultaneously moving toward the body you desire so deeply in your mind. Nobody said you had to choose. You get to save up for the new car, while still rocking out, and getting from point A to point B, in the car you have today. Wanting a new car does not have to take away from the fact that you have a car that runs today.

Some of us may also believe that acceptance can cultivate laziness. Clients in the past have told me that hating their body motivated them to eat healthy and exercise, that if they didn't hate their body, they would lie around eating pints of ice cream every day. This fear is very real, but completely inaccurate.

It is true that initial motivation, for most people, comes from moving away from what they don't want. It's a good initial push to get moving. However, if you keep facing the direction of what you don't want, and walking backward toward what you do want, you will always be facing the wrong direction, and you will likely never achieve what you desire. It's your job, at some point, to turn around and move toward what you do want—facing forward. This is the only effective long-term strategy.

Many of us also believe that we have to work extremely hard to get results. We have to pour our blood, sweat, and tears into whatever we're doing, otherwise it's worthless. From this mindset, we believe that if we are simply accepting ourselves and enjoying life, change can't possibly occur! And so the type of weight loss described in this book might sound too simple. Often times, however, it is that simple.

If you are working really hard at something and you continue running into the same wall over and over, what you're doing is not right for you. The goal isn't right or your approach isn't right. Your blood, sweat, and tears are coming from running into a wall over and over. You may feel validated in your work ethic, but you are not getting anywhere. It's time to go around the wall instead of attempting to force your way through it. It will feel simple in comparison to pushing through bricks, but it's no less valid.

Move toward simplicity and move toward forgiveness—forgiveness for gaining weight in the first place. For stuffing down the emotions and checking out. For going numb with food or technology.

The truth is you are more than just a body. You have a core self and are an amazing person. You have a shell with skin, bones, fat, and muscle, but what's really inside of this shell? What about your shell says anything about who you are?

One very important shift that needs to happen in order to lose weight and accept yourself is to picture your ideal body and life. It's powerful to dream and vision first. You may want to wait for the scale to go down or "see it to believe it." However, it's more effective to see the numbers go down, to see your ideal life and your ideal body, in your head, first. Visioning enables your subconscious to see where you want to go, which makes it easier for it to take you there.

Remember we spoke earlier about a potential fear of the unknown. Visioning allows this dream life to be less of an unknown because your subconscious has actually experienced it. It shifts from a distant dream and quickly becomes a simple destination you typed into your GPS.

Your subconscious communicates with pictures, senses, and feelings. When you are visioning, be in the moment. See what's around you. Feel, smell, and taste your surroundings. Allow that vision to feel real—to be more pronounced than your fears. In those moments of panic, when your confidence is weary, it's your vision that will pull you through and help you receive everything you desire.

Questions for Transformation:

1. **What's keeping me from accepting my current body as I move toward what I desire?** Get honest with yourself here. What fears are lurking behind acceptance, and are they accurate? What real, concrete evidence do you have that accepting yourself today will grant you something other than everything you desire? You've most likely never truly tried this strategy.

2. **What does my ideal body look like, feel like?** This is visionary work. Who is around you? Where you are standing? Get in touch with all of your deepest desires and connect with them as much as possible, using all of your senses. See this vision as your inevitable destination. Believe it and expect it.

3. **What feelings have I decided I will feel once I lose weight?**

More happiness? Confidence? Radiance? Write them all down and ask yourself how you might achieve these feelings today. If your current body was your body for life, and there was nothing you could do to change it physically, how would you attain these feelings?

4. **What morning routine can I add to increase and show gratitude toward what I currently love about my body and life?** How can you create powerful and inspiring mornings to set off your day?

Step Two: Honor Time

In the financial world, it is said that a person's bank account will tell you exactly what the person prioritizes. In other words, if every person on the planet had the same exact income, they would all spend it differently. The way in which we spend our money highlights what we believe is important or necessary to invest in.

We may not all have the exact same income, but we do share a common account. We all have exactly 24 hours each day. Time is as much of a resource as money. And, just as with money, we all choose to spend our time differently.

Some of us work more. Some sleep more. Some of us have lots of down time, and some hardly have any at all. The way in which you are filling your time will directly reflect the way in which you live your life, in the same way that the way you spend your money will.

If you spend your money on a lot of stuff, you will have a lot of stuff, but perhaps not a lot of money. If you invest your money in things that create more wealth, you may have less stuff but more money. Eventually, you may choose to spend that extra money on more stuff. Personally, I like to do both. I choose to invest a large portion of my money in things that create more wealth, and I also like to buy things that bring me joy in this moment. I recommend doing the same with your time.

Many people believe they have to sacrifice a lot right now, in order to have a satisfying life in later years. An example is the person who works long hours six days a week in order to save for retirement, where he won't have to work anymore. I've never bought in to this way of thinking. To me, it's always made more sense to work a balanced amount of time now so that I don't have to put my life on hold until retirement. However, I also spend my working time on things I enjoy, which makes it easier to decide that I don't want to stop working unless I have to stop.

Consider how this might relate to your body. Are you spending all of your time on activities that are counterproductive to your best body and life, perhaps with the hope that at some point you can live an alternate way that is more aligned with what you desire? If so, how do you feel in the present moment? If you're putting all of your time into a bunch of work (a diet) so that you can retire (stop dieting and be thin), you're feeling stressed, tired, and overwhelmed. Does this sound like an effective strategy for living your best life?

Doesn't it make more sense to make our current lives, the present day we have, as close as possible to our ideal lives? Meaning, if we don't picture ourselves spending time weighing out food, counting calories, and living as a slave to the gym when we are in our ideal body, then it isn't an effective way to achieve that body. Instead, we should map out the life we want to live once we're in our ideal body and just begin living that life now.

The way in which you spend your time is more of your choice than you may believe. It takes planning and prioritizing to create a body and life you love, just as it takes planning and prioritizing to create the wealth you desire. When we live truthfully, we spend our time on the things that are in alignment with our ideal body and life.

This means we can't wake up and go along with the motions. We can't show up at a job we hate each and every day, counting down the days to the weekend. We must take deliberate action to make time for the activities that come naturally and feel good so that we can be the true version of ourselves.

I realize that not everyone has total flexibility to walk away from some of the less-than-ideal activities on which they spend their time. It isn't necessary to eliminate every activity you don't enjoy. What is necessary is to acknowledge how you currently spend your time and how you ideally would like to spend your time, and then create a plan to better blend these two worlds.

When I ask my clients what they will do once they retire or what they'd do if they won millions of dollars and never had to work again, many of them say they'd travel. And, while there are some people who truly do want to hop in an RV or plane and travel for years around the world, the majority of my clients are simply craving more fun and relaxation than they currently have in their lives. "Travel" becomes the catch-all activity for that fun and relaxation.

But we don't have to travel around the world to experience the benefits of travel. Most of us can gain the same benefits from a few short trips a couple of times a year, as long as we fill up our everyday lives with fun, relaxation, and adventure, too. So when you're planning your ideal activities, don't go with the automatic response. Instead, think on what would make your life truly better. How do you really want to spend your time?

When our days are more closely aligned with our ideal body and life, we begin to step into that body and life. Therefore, if you see yourself being more social and getting involved in more adventures and activities once you have your ideal body, then it's time to add that in your life now. It cannot afford to wait until your body is smaller. It absolutely must begin now.

If you're having trouble envisioning how you truly want to spend your time, a good place to start is by identifying your natural gifts. Are you good with the arts, mechanics, building, or caring? If you aren't sure, look into your past. What games did you play as a kid? Did you play teacher, house, cops and robbers, tag, or video games? What did your life look like as a kid and what does that say about you today? I loved arts and crafts, and I was always looking for Crayola's new thing. That says a lot about who I am because creativity is a huge part of my life, and without it I couldn't be me.

Who are you when nobody is around? When I ask people what they are good at I get responses like, "I am a good friend, mother, wife," or "I make people laugh." But what about when nobody is there? It's great that you are a giver and a great friend, but who are you *really*? Who were you throughout your life? What do you do for fun? What are your hobbies?

What hobbies did you stop doing? We tend to have more hobbies in adolescence, but then drop them as we get busy and take on more responsibilities. I assure you your body knows this. It remembers everything, and it definitely knows what brings you happiness and that it isn't part of your life anymore. Your body knows if you found joy from a sport your whole life and then all of a sudden stopped playing. If you stopped playing soccer because you don't have a team to play with, at least do something that resembles soccer. Find something through which your body can release its desire for soccer.

After you look into all the things you are naturally inclined to do, begin to look at all the things you have always wanted to do. What do you want to try? What have you been too scared to try? Maybe you try yoga, geology, dancing, or guitar lessons. Trying something new can instill a great deal of confidence. It also reminds us that skills are always available to be learned. As mentioned, living naturally thin is simply a skillset to be learned. So as you learn a new activity, you will begin to see how capable you are of learning anything, even being naturally thin.

As children, we often hear words of praise and encouragement said in a way that detracts from the time it took to build a skill. For example, I will watch my son attempt to put a puzzle piece in his puzzle several times before he actually gets it in the appropriate spot. When he does this he looks at me for encouragement.

If I tell him, "Great job!" I am instilling confidence, but I am taking away from the fact that it took him several tries to accomplish this task. His brain remembers the praise, and links it to the puzzle piece fitting in. Later in life, he may have a desire to learn a new skill and think back to the times he received praise. He may forget that it took him an hour to get in that puzzle piece and assume that any new skill should be easily learned. He may assume that if the skill is not easily learned, perhaps it's not a skill he's good at.

This is inaccurate thinking. We have to remember that we learned how to do all the things we do. We just forget about the time and practice it took for many of them. We don't remember how many times we fell before we crawled or walked. We just remember that we did it.

If it is something we enjoy, we forget all the effort it took to master it because it didn't seem like work. It seemed like fun. And so, when we go to learn something new that isn't as enjoyable, but is perhaps necessary, we hyper-focus on the fact that we're not getting it right away. Then we jump to conclusions about what that means about us. In many cases, we stop trying.

To counter-act this, I don't simply tell my son, "Great job!" Instead, I say, "You got the puzzle piece in because you kept trying!" This reminds him that the effort he put in is what is being praised, not the fact that he completed the task.

We literally can accomplish anything we desire. Luckily,

we don't desire everything, which makes it easier to make choices on how we choose to spend our time. I have no desire to be an astronaut or to learn how to crochet. And so I don't have to spend any time learning those skills. But I do desire many other things that I don't currently know how to do, and I expect time will be needed to master them. In fact, the further away these skills are from my current skills, the harder they will be to master. But that doesn't mean that I am not good at them. It just means I haven't learned them yet.

As humans, we seek adventure. It's a part of who we are. When we don't get it, we feel as though something is missing. So plan your travels each year but also make the most of your current time, in the city in which you live.

When you're at home, challenge yourself to ask what you want to do before you automatically eat or watch television. When you're in your city, explore before deciding on a restaurant or activity. Spend your time with as much joy, fun, creativity, and adventure as possible. Then when you crave a Netflix binge, you will enjoy every minute of it.

Exercises for Transformation:

1. Make a list of past hobbies or activities that you have stopped doing and would like to do again. Prioritize and plan your time to include more of these in your life right now and in the future.

2. Make a list of how you currently spend your time. Account for all 24 hours. Don't forget about grooming, eating, cooking, driving, etc. Figure out where all of your time goes and then ask yourself if this is how you want to spend your time. If not, how can you adjust it?

3. Make a list of new hobbies or activities that you would like to try. Think of everything you say you would like to do, except you're not good at. Make time to try it anyway. If you have the desire to do it, you can do it.

Live Abundantly

An important distinction between the naturally thin and those who battle weight is the idea of abundance versus dearth. The naturally thin have no reason to believe that any food is off limits, as they believe they can eat what they want and remain thin. They quite literally can have their cake and eat it, too. Due to this belief, food is in complete abundance to them, making it seemingly boring. For the dieters of the world, food is anything but abundant. Entire food groups are labeled as "off-limits," making food in general a deprivation.

This creates a major issue for your body and your brain. A study done by Wood in 2001 found that dieting dropped levels of leptin by 54 percent, which increases hunger. They also found that the desire to eat doubled after three months of dieting. Hart and Chiovari found that dieting causes an increase in obsessive thoughts around food. And Rogerson, Soltani, and Copeland found that dieting leads to increase of appetite, food obsessions, and increased cravings.

Even though food is actually available in large amounts, when you diet you live as though you are on a deserted island, scouring for the last bite of food. No wonder you can't stop thinking about your next meal all day long!

Food becomes an obsession because your mind feels deprived of it constantly. You are constantly making lists of all the foods you cannot eat, or can only eat in "moderation." You're focused on the lack of what you want, not on what you want. And this doesn't just happen with food.

Anytime you utter the sentence, "I didn't get enough ..." you are placing yourself in a world of lack and deprivation. You may wake up and say you didn't get enough sleep, and then go to bed saying, "I didn't get enough done today." You complain about not having enough time, money, or fun. And all these declarations of not enough add up to a life of lack in which you're always hungry for the things and food you believe you can't have.

Total Body Transformation:

If you want to transform your body, the task here is quite simple: Stop dieting. Food has to become available in any type or amount. This doesn't mean that you need to eat an entire cake, but it does mean that a cake everyday needs to be an option in your mind. Only when you have the option, do you gift your mind the ability to truly make a choice, to say "I don't want cake everyday" instead of "I can't have cake everyday." One statement comes from a place of choice and abundance. The other comes from a place of deprivation.

The linguistics may seem silly, but the impact is profound. You cannot transform your body into its ideal form when you make it live from a place of fear and scarcity. The minute you step out of deprivation around food, you step into freedom and choice.

Keep in mind that some foods will trigger negative reactions in your body: digestive upset, heartburn, and/or sluggishness. You may also have food allergies or be diabetic. The language you use around these foods is still crucial. You still must switch your thoughts from "can't have" to "choose not to have."

It is always your choice. You *can* eat sugar as a diabetic, but the results aren't pleasant. I *can* eat large amounts of dairy, but the consequences—to me—aren't worth it. You must eliminate the language of lack from your vocabulary and realize that thin people eat an assortment of all kinds of foods. Some eat dairy. Some do not. Some eat lots of sugar. Some hardly at all. There is no one type of eating style that leads to thin, only the eating style that fits you best. And, for every thin person, it's a different style of eating.

Your job is to figure out what types of foods make you feel best and to stay away from extremes. Many people who struggle with weight say things like, "Well, thin people just have everything in moderation." This is technically true, but the statement is still inaccurate because it's not how thin people describe how they eat.

The naturally thin say they just eat everything. They may naturally eat less sugar than the person who is dieting, but not with any conscious effort. They just reach for the foods that sound good to them. This is what you are learning to do as well. Don't state in advance how much sugar you are *allowed* to eat. Instead, consciously decide how much you want to eat, in the moment, in a way that still feels good in your body and life.

Total Life Transformation:

To transform more than just your body, you must go beyond moving away from deprivation and start looking at the quality of your food and life. This is the difference between a person who is thin and unhappy and the person who is thin and truly thriving in life. There are plenty of people who are alive, but how many of them are truly living?

Step One: Prioritize Quality of Food

It is my belief that all food is created equal until it feels bad in your body. In other words, no food is bad in any way until your body gives you a negative reaction. This reaction could be described as low quality *for you*. This requires you to remove the judgment before you eat something. Every day is different, and every day may require different foods or amounts from you.

If you eat fast food and notice that every time you eat it you have a negative reaction, you probably will want to remove that food from your diet most of the time. Having said that, if you choose to eat it anyway, then you are choosing a low-quality lunch and a low-quality afternoon. This is fine; you don't need to judge yourself if that is your choice, but just know that that's what you are choosing for that day and remove the negative voices that like to follow these decisions.

A client of mine used to show up to his workouts every Friday morning with low energy, feeling sluggish. It wasn't typical for him to be so tired, and I noticed it was consistent. It happened every Friday. Finally I asked him, "What did you eat this morning for breakfast?"

He told me that on Friday mornings he had an appointment before our session that required him to wake up earlier so he would grab a breakfast sandwich at a fast food restaurant. Without judgment, I reminded him that a breakfast of that quality would affect his workout negatively. I also reminded him that he paid for our sessions so it was completely his choice what he wanted to receive from each of them.

He stated that the workouts always felt so hard on Fridays and therefore requested we brainstorm some breakfast alternatives. I recommended stopping at a local shop that makes healthy smoothies or even grabbing a bagel sandwich from a higher quality restaurant. He thought about it and proceeded to say that he would prefer to simply wake up earlier and make the breakfast he truly enjoyed.

After making that simple change for many weeks in a row, he reported that he couldn't believe what a difference it made in his workout and overall energy. He never imagined one breakfast sandwich could have such an impact on his day. He never had problems with Friday morning workouts again.

Note that I never once told him not to eat the fast food sandwich. I simply reminded him of the consequences of eating it and asked whether or not he felt it was worth it. If he was going to be lying around all day, eating a fast food sandwich may be appropriate. But he wanted to be productive. If you want to be productive, eating poorly can pose a challenge to accomplishing what you truly desire.

As mentioned earlier, people of all shapes and sizes eat all sorts of foods. Fast food is not just reserved for the fat people of the world. This means you need to be careful of your judgments. The next time you judge someone or yourself, remember that it's not the food itself that causes problems for you or this person.

People struggling with weight can eat as many pieces of cake as they want, because their excess weight has nothing to do with the actual piece of cake. It is how we eat the cake that makes a difference in our digestion, metabolism, and ultimately our weight. This is why you must take judgment off yourself and other people with food.

As I have mentioned in previous steps, you must live in your ideal body now if you wish to reach your weight-loss goals. This means you must eat like you have your ideal body now. If that includes cake, eat up!

At one of my events, one of the attendees said she really wanted a Milk Dud but felt guilty for wanting one. When I asked her why she felt guilty about having a milk-dud desire, she said, "I don't need a Milk Dud, it's just extra calories. It's not going to give me energy, and it's probably not good for me."

These sound like valid answers to most people. And most people would have told her to be strong and hold off from the Milk Duds. However, I do things differently. I asker her, "If you were 130 pounds, would you eat some Milk Duds?"

She replied, "Hell yeah, I would. If I was 130 pounds, I couldn't care less."

This was a huge shift for her, but it's the correct answer. If you intend to eat Milk Duds at your goal weight, you better start enjoying them now! Otherwise, you are telling your body that you are doing something one way, and then changing it later. If you do that, your body won't give you the same reaction.

Most people don't actually believe that when they reach their goal weight they are going to be overeating, binge eating, fast-food junkies, or anything close to that. In fact, most people describe their ideal body and life as a very balanced style of eating and exercising. So why not begin eating the way you would like to eat the rest of your life now?

Plenty of people eat crappy food and don't gain weight. Others eat all organic with no carbohydrates and struggle with an excess 60 pounds. It isn't about what they're eating. It's how they're eating it.

The thin person who eats low-quality food but doesn't gain weight has no negative emotion toward that food. This may not be a good thing, as low-quality food can still lead to an unhealthy internal system—even in the thin—but that reaction is not going on their body. It's going *into* it. If you are someone who wears every negative reaction toward food on your stomach, you will probably strive to remove those habits that cause the negative reactions *by choice*. This is a healthy thing.

Just to clarify, thin people may have reactions to low-quality food, but their bodies don't use weight gain as a way to communicate this. This means it's possible that it doesn't matter how much crappy food they eat, they won't gain weight, but they still may harm their bodies. They just respond differently.

If I put anything in my body that it doesn't like, I get a storm of negative responses. Sometimes this can be annoying, because I just want to eat some food, and I can't without my body getting furious. As annoying as this is, however, it's actually a good thing! These reactions mean my body and my mind are in alignment and practicing great communication. If you aren't experiencing these reactions, eat what you want. If it's low quality, just make sure you remove the judgment. Maybe it isn't the best decision, but it's the decision you have made in that moment. Own it, and move on.

Removing the judgment removes the fear, which releases you from weight gain. People who are naturally thin have a much smaller fear of weight gain than those who struggle with their weight. In my research, over 50 percent of the ideal-weight participants reported no fear of weight gain, while only one percent of overweight participants said the same. When asked how food impacts their life, ideal-weight participants stated that it impacts it positively through pleasure and enjoyment, while overweight participants stated their top response to food as emotional distress.

Food doesn't cause weight gain. Your thoughts do. When you continuously ignore your negative reactions or attach negative emotion to your body's reactions, you gain weight. When you release these negative reactions and emotions, you release the weight gain.

Sometimes I just really want a scoop of ice cream. I don't feel negative toward this decision even though I know the ice cream will make my stomach hurt. If I want it enough to put up with my body's response, I eat it, and I don't judge myself for doing it. I also don't gain weight from it.

The distinction here is noticing when your body is giving you a physical negative reaction, and, when your mind is giving you judgment and shame. The latter is dysfunctional for living in your ideal body.

Your body is smart. This is why food that causes a stomachache or heartburn can be eliminated out of your body, by your body. If you want your body to eliminate the food that is not serving you, you must let go of your mind's negative reactions around that food. Brush the reaction off, and let your body eliminate that food for you. This process of elimination will happen without force by you, so relax and allow your body to automatically get rid of that food that isn't serving you.

When you release the guilt and shame and let your body pick your foods for you, you will find that it gravitates toward high-quality foods. This is natural and important. When you feed yourself high-quality food, you are saying that you deserve self-care and self- love. You are saying that you—and your body—are worth the best. A fine restaurant or a great home-cooked meal supports these beliefs far more than fast food.

When you eat at a nice restaurant, the chefs use their creativity to put flavors and foods together while making the plate look beautiful. A nice restaurant also has optimal lighting and relaxing or enjoyable music. The atmosphere enables you to truly enjoy the food that has been made with so much love, thought, and care. This is a high-quality experience and your body responds well to it.

Your own home-cooked food will be even higher quality because you are putting your love, thought, and care into it. That's the best you can get, and your body will respond to your efforts.

Note: Throwing something into the microwave doesn't count. This may be food made at home but it isn't full of love and care. It's easy and thought-free. When you serve your body pre-packaged food, you are saying you—and it— are not worth the time it takes to prepare and cook a nice meal.

When you prepare food for yourself (or have someone prepare it for you), you are putting time and preparation into it, which equals love and abundance. It takes time and planning to put together high-quality food for you and your loved ones. It takes high-quality ingredients and love to plate nutritious and delicious foods.

This means that as much as possible, you want to avoid all those short cuts. Prepared foods are easier and they save time, and there are times when they are totally appropriate. But those times ideally won't be all of the time. Not only will eating packaged food feel worse to your body, your mind will likely also feel worse. You'll feel less fulfilled at the mealtimes when you are simply heating something up. There is something special about you taking the time to put high-quality ingredients together, and then sitting down and enjoying the fruits of your labor.

Keeping with this theory, fast food becomes kind of insane. There is no care, no thought, and no love put into this type of food. It is slapped together by people who probably don't want to be there. The food is frozen to save time. It has preservatives to save money, and it is all about making it faster and easier to serve and eat. This creates a less en-joyable meal for you, and a low-quality food source for your body. Of course, there are times when this is an appropriate option, but how often are you relying on this, instead of tak-ing the time and care your food really deserves?

The story you tell yourself about not having enough time or money to eat high-quality foods comes from your habitual pattern of lack. As long as you continue to tell yourself you lack what you need to eat well, you will live that lack. If you don't have a lot of time, find the time you do have, and de-vote that time to meal planning and prep so that cooking becomes faster and easier.

You can purchase services to help you with this. You could

hire a private chef to cook your meals or prep all your meals for the week. You can use one of the countless meal prep services that ship all the ingredients and recipes to your door, where all you have to do is cook it. Or, my favorite, you can utilize a meal planning site that tells you what to cook each night, gives you your grocery list, and lists all of your prep.

If you don't have a lot of money, purchase the highest quality ingredients you can, within your budget, or grow what you can. You may need to prioritize your money differently to increase your food quality, but this is not an area I recommend skimping on. Look at your budget each month and ask yourself, "Where is my money going that I could move to our grocery bill?"

Questions for Transformation:

1. **Is it time to stop dieting for good?** This is the time to make a real decision and finally divorce dieting for good. If that feels overwhelming then at least take a 14-day break from dieting and reassess at that time.

2. **How do I see myself eating in my ideal body and life?** Be really honest with yourself in how you would like to experience food. You design your life however you'd like. Then begin taking steps to live that way now.

3. **What is stopping me from eating that way today?** The thoughts that come up around this are often limiting beliefs and are not true. Food is not the problem, so begin eating the way you would like to forever.

4. **What steps do I need to take to make my life feel more abundant?** Look at your linguistic patterns around lack (when you say "not enough") and also look at the things and places where you feel deprived.

5. **How can I begin increasing the quality of my food right now?** Look at the limiting beliefs and excuses that are get-

ting in the way of you eating the kinds of foods you deserve.

Step Two: Emphasize Quality of Life

I've mentioned before that the mind prefers consistency. Therefore, change can feel scary and threatening to a perceived calm and event-free mental state. And so this intention to make changes causes your mind to play a trick on you that directly impacts your quality of life.

If you look back, you'll notice there have been times in your life when you've had glimpses of your utmost desires. Those desires felt real and true for you, albeit, perhaps, far away. You may think about this dream life the way one would of unicorns and fairies, but it continues to make appearances throughout your lifetime, trying to seduce you toward it. Most of the time, however, you push it down and away, convinced you can't attain it.

Then, when things get really bad—the scale reaches a new high, the doctor threatens you with a health condition, your entire wardrobe stops fitting—you make a powerful decision to change, to move toward that dream life. And with your best foot forward, you begin making all sorts of changes to achieve your desires, with motivation and inspiration guiding you. But then, you lose your motivation to continue with these changes and your body and life go back to where they were, sometimes even farther from where you wanted to be.

Once that happens, you are defeated and frustrated. You believe you'll never achieve your dream life, and so you grudgingly settle for where you are. And your dream wanders back off into the distance.

It doesn't have to be this way, but you must understand how the mind works to avoid this. When you start making changes, your brain plays a trick that convinces you that your old life, the one far away from your dream life, is not that bad. Your brain says it is okay to settle. You hear yourself say things like, "It could be worse" or "Life isn't so bad."

The longer you settle, the longer your previous low point becomes your current set point. You continue to drift farther and farther away from your dream life, and so it becomes increasingly less attainable, until it permanently fixates itself as nothing more than a dream. Your toleration ceiling moves farther and farther up, enabling you to tolerate far more than you were ever meant to tolerate.

Your job is to wake up and notice this trick. Settling for anything less than what you truly desire is not a way to live. It's not to say that everything you desire needs to come to fruition in this moment, but it is imperative that you continuously move toward it, every single day. To live a high-quality life, you must refuse to stay stuck in a life you don't love.

You need to go after the money you want, the relationship you want, the body you want, and eliminate anything that gets in the way. Remember: My personal belief is if you can desire it, you can have it. I believe that's why we don't desire everything. This allows everything you desire to be attainable. Why else would you have glimpses of your dream life? Assuming they are true, your desires come from you. Therefore, I believe, you have the tools necessary to achieve them.

All it takes is creative problem solving and resourcefulness. In general terms, men tend to have an easier time compartmentalizing. Men tend to be equipped with the ability to state a desire, decide on a course of action, and then attain their desire while keeping the heaviness of life separate. For example, when couples lose weight together, the men usually lose weight each week, while the women flounder, disgruntled by their husbands' easy results. The thought processes are usually very different between these two genders.

Men tend to say, "I want to lose weight." Then they decide on a strategy, like cutting calories or spending an hour each day at the gym, and they just do it. That's the whole process. Just as they may say, "I want to make a million dollars," decide on a strategy, and move on to achieving it.

Women, in general, tend to start off the same, but then when it comes to applying the strategy, a whole mess of stuff gets in the way. They bring years of failure into the mix, with baggage from childhood experiences and emotions like judgment, shame, and insecurity so their results are all over the place.

Compartmentalizing is the right approach for attaining your dream life. You still want to acknowledge your emotions as you move forward toward your goals, but keep them separate from your results. Yes, you have emotions about your weight, but they have nothing to do with your ability to follow steps toward learning a new skill. Your mind has blended them, and your job now is to keep them separate. If you let them blend together, your problem-solving abilities are lowered and your resourcefulness is eliminated.

Let's use a money example. Let's say you need $5,000 to invest in yourself to achieve your best life. You really believe this money will help you get unstuck and receive the skills you need to achieve everything you desire. But you don't have that money in your bank account in this moment. Most people would simply say, "I don't have the money," feel sad about it, and move on, still stuck in their current circumstances. Then, as time passed, they would forget about the opportunity to change their life, and everything would stay the same because they already decided it was okay to settle.

But what if I approached you with a check for $10,000 and told you I really needed $5,000 right now, and that if you could give it to me today then I would give you this $10,000 check to cash in five days? Would you say, "Sorry, I don't have it," or would you find a way to come up with the funds so you could make $5,000 in five days?

Most people say they would try their hardest to come up with that $5,000 in one day in order to get the check for $10,000. They would max out their credit cards, ask people for money, sell stuff, or do whatever it takes. In other words, they would get resourceful. But there is no emotional baggage on coming up with money to cash a check in a few days for more money. It's very matter of fact, so your creative thinking and resourcefulness are at their peak.

But when it comes to investing $5,000 in yourself—your very best investment—the creative thinking and resourcefulness are long gone. Now you are worrying about whether or not you can succeed since you've failed so many times in the past. You think about how far away this dream life is from where you are. You wonder if you're worth it, if you can do it. You decide you aren't or that you can't, and your mind—that mind that prefers congruence and consistency—tells you that settling for the life you have isn't so bad. And so you stay stuck. Without the guarantee of a return on investment, you're unwilling to take the risk.

This is a mistake.

I read a story that Mark Zuckerberg, the CEO of Facebook, invited a handful of friends to his dorm room to discuss his new idea and present an investment opportunity. Only two people showed up to this meeting and took immediate action. Now both of those men are billionaires. The other people made excuses as to why they couldn't make the meeting. When an opportunity presents itself, take a risk, and receive the reward.

You can't move forward toward your dreams without taking a risk. You just can't. If you go through life searching for guarantees you will only receive what you can guarantee: for everything to stay the same or get worse.

To have a high-quality life, you must be willing to take risks, especially on yourself. Worst-case scenario is that you walk away with an important lesson, which means at least you tried. If you sit back and wish for things to change, they won't. If you are out there trying things, taking risks, and open to the possibility of success or failure, your life will continue to move forward. And eventually, it will all click. You will find the right resource or creatively solve a problem in the most productive of ways, and everything you desire will show up. Usually, at this point, all the past risks you took will become useful and helpful to your new breakthrough, and you'll realize nothing was a waste at all.

Theodore Roosevelt said: "The credit belongs to the man who is actually in the arena, whose face is marred by dust and sweat and blood; who strives valiantly; who errs, who comes short again and again, because there is no effort without errors and shortcoming; but who does actually strive to do the deeds; who knows great enthusiasms, the great devotions; who spends himself in a worthy cause; who at the best knows in the end the triumph of high achievement, and who at the worst, if he fails, at least fails while daring greatly, so that his place shall never be with those cold and timid souls who neither know victory nor defeat."

Not knowing defeat may feel like a noble way to live your life, but it eliminates the possibility of victory. Choosing not to take risks anymore due to too many rounds in the arena may feel like the safest way to live, but it only moves you backward, away from what you truly desire. You must be willing to get back in the arena until you find the solutions you are looking for and the life you really want.

Become addicted to solutions. Train yourself to see roadblocks as nothing more than opportunities to find new solutions or to problem solve differently. When I first had major digestive issues, I got super curious and went into problem solving mode. I didn't settle and say, "Well I guess this is just how I feel when I eat," and then take a drug to mask the symptoms. I searched furiously for solutions, and I found them. But I didn't always live this way. I used to settle for the life I was handed instead of going after the life I wanted.

Now I believe there is a solution for everything. There are all types of experts out there who have mastered something that you are currently struggling with. There are creative people that have invented products and services that solve a problem you have right now. And, if there isn't, there is always the potential for you to be exactly the person to create that solution and market it to the world for the others who need it.

Refuse to settle. Envision your dream life, and creatively solve problems to get there. Never stop searching for the solutions to create exactly what you desire. Never be afraid to get back in the arena.

Questions for Transformation:

1. **How am I currently settling?** What are you aware of in this moment that doesn't make you happy? What do you simply tolerate? List all these tolerations.

2. **What is my dream life?** What does your life look like without all of these tolerations? What do you truly desire without holding back at all?

3. **What do I perceive are the obstacles that are in the way of attaining my dream life?** What's getting in the way of your creative problem solving and resourcefulness?

4. **What are some changes I can make in this moment to move closer to my dream life?** What feels possible right now? What risks do you need to take to make these changes possible? Remember, a risk could be emotional. For example, you could risk failing and feeling defeated. But, you could also get everything you desire and more.

5. **What solutions do I need to find?** Where are you hitting a problem-solving wall? Where do you need to search for solutions outside of yourself? State your exact need, and the solution will show up.

6. **Who do I need to hire or what products/services do I**

need to purchase to support my journey to attaining my dream life? Once you decide where you need additional solutions, opportunities to invest in these solutions may show up. Which are available now? Are there some that you want to find?

Live Deliciously

Nearly everyone enjoys food. The tastes, textures, and smells are sensory pleasures in which we all revel. For dieters, however, food has become something other than a pleasurable experience that satisfies hunger and nourishes the body. Instead, it has become the cause of their weight. It is something they put into their bodies that doesn't leave in the ways they would like. Instead, it hangs around as excess weight, which turns food—a pleasurable thing—into a negative.

Total Body Transformation:

To transform your body, you simply need to find ways in which you can enable the body to burn the fat it doesn't need rather than to store it. You may believe that your body cannot do this, because of past experiences, or you may believe that you have to follow some trick or try a gimmick to make this happen. I disagree.

I do not believe there is anything special you have to do to switch from storing to burning fat other than to recognize that's what's happening in your body right now and then get out of your body's way.

Your body is designed to burn the fat it doesn't need. At some point, your belief systems overrode that physical system. This most likely happened for a good reason. You may have been too stressed, or too overwhelmed, and living in survival for some reason or another. And so you took over the system and the body obeyed. **It stored the fat as future reserves, because you told it you needed more of something.**

Now, though, it's time to hand the reins back to your body. Let the body do what it already knows how to do. Go busy yourself elsewhere with joy, fulfillment, fun, and deliciousness. Tell your body you have enough, *show* your body you have enough, and it will release what you don't need.

I believe a body that is ideal experiences a lot of pleasure, and food is meant to be pleasurable. In fact, that's how I was brought up, and my family doesn't struggle with obesity. We were taught that you should cook your meals with the freshest ingredients because they will taste the best. We were taught to enjoy the pleasures of food and were never forced to clean our plates. We were shown a healthy, positive relationship with food, which enabled us to feel we always had enough.

I talk about food in almost every one of my steps because food wears so many hats. Food is highly emotional and can play a role in many aspects of your life. However, this step is about macronutrient balance and discussing how to have a healthy relationship with food like the one I had growing up as a child.

Most of you know the major macronutrients: proteins, carbohydrates, and fats. It is my belief that all of these are created equal. This doesn't mean I want you to count grams and make sure they are equal. It means that all three are positive and good for you until you find a negative response. For example, you don't need to cut carbohydrates out of your diet unless every time you eat carbohydrates you fall asleep, as that would be a negative reaction.

Some people do have bad reactions to carbohydrates so

of course they would want to choose something else that doesn't cause adverse reactions. There are also people out there who simply have preferences. Maybe you don't like protein or meat sources so you eat less of them. That doesn't mean there is something wrong with you or that you are going to gain weight. You could love avocados and olive oil, and maybe have more fat in your diet than someone else, but this still doesn't mean you are going to gain weight.

It always comes back to how you feel. We have been conditioned to believe that carbohydrates are the devil so your mind could tell you to feel guilty. We are told, "You can't eat the bread and pasta because that's too many carbohydrates." If you feel great after the bread and pasta, then eat up! Don't worry about combinations, percentages, or grams unless you are an athlete or in competitive sports.

How do you feel after eating bread and pasta? I myself would be too full if I ate both together, and I love pasta a lot more than bread, so I would skip the bread to leave room for the pasta that I desire so much. If I really wanted bread I might order something lighter so I could still enjoy it. At the end of the day, we only have so much appetite. Knowing what we want—and honoring that—is the key to a healthy relationship with food.

Keep in mind I am speaking in terms of weight loss only. If you know you don't do well with that many carbohydrates from a medical perspective, you probably want to listen to that. But allow yourself to choose not to eat them, as opposed to stating that you cannot or should not eat them. Using "can't" or "shouldn't" language puts food into the deprivation category, which interferes with your ability to choose not to eat it.

If you are a competitive body builder, understanding your macronutrients is very important. But, if you are just going on with your merry day it won't matter. If you are eating too much or too little of any nutrient, your body will always tell you. Here are some easy signs to look for:

Too little carbohydrates = low energy, mood swings

Too little protein = really weak, don't put on muscle

Too little fat = hair falling out, nails are brittle

These are just some reactions your body can give you. You could look up each one of these to learn more about each nutrient and what it does for your body, if you want. Remember, though, that you don't have to be an athlete. Just eat in a way that makes you feel good. You're not running a marathon tomorrow!

Total Life Transformation:

I mentioned in previous steps the importance of cooking your own food there so that there is more love, care, and thought which equals more enjoyment and fulfillment. If you would like to receive those benefits, allow your body to look at food without judgment and feel the reactions.

Don't worry about calories; just do what feels good. Naturally thin people may still overeat, but they don't have guilt. In fact, the vast majority of them couldn't tell you how many calories they eat in any given day. What they usually say is that they eat when they are hungry and stop when they are full. They still have times of over indulgence or gluttony. They just assume their body will handle it.

Be aware, too, of where your decisions around food come from. Many are likely vanity-related, not health-related. Let's be honest, if our entire society thought only in terms of health, we would live in a completely different world. It's really not about health entirely, which is why people who eat unhealthy food and are thin don't have guilt. People might think, *If I could eat fast food every day and stay thin that would be great.* But these thin people may actually be unhealthy. Still, no one judges them because, in general, our society cares only about what we see with our eyes.

To transform your life, start focusing on health and what feels good, and be careful how you judge thin people. For all you know, they could have horrible diets; they just don't have guilt or a negative relationship with food so they don't gain weight.

Being someone who has lived naturally thin, overweight, and thin again, this was the biggest difference to me. When reflecting back and looking at the difference between my two bodies I noticed that when I was thin I just wasn't thinking about it. It didn't matter what I ate because I had so many other things to think about. Food provided me pleasure and that was the end of it. Of course, there were times when I overate. I would think, *Oh, this pizza is so good! I'm going to have another slice.* And so I ate it.

It never occurred to me that what I ate affected my weight so if I wanted another slice, why not? This is what I want for you. Can you imagine what your life would look life if you adopted that belief?

The French culture doesn't have everything perfect, but the culture as a whole has a very different approach to weight than we do. They are big on long, savory meals. They're also big on long, savory lives.

Here in the United States we don't have three-hour meals, and we focus on results at the gym, whether that's rock hard abs or toned thighs. The French don't have three-hour meals every meal, but they have them often, and French women savor their bodies. They don't need to be rock hard; they don't over exercise in the gym. They savor life by dressing up just because it makes them feel good. They don't need a reason. They just do things for themselves. They savor movement very differently than we do, too. They walk and take stairs as a way of life, not out of force.

I am not saying that we need to become French, but we can

take away nuggets of wisdom like slowing down, removing guilt, doing things for ourselves, and eliminating our obsession with having a rock-hard body.

This obsession with rock-hard bodies seems to be an American obsession, and it usually comes from other women. Trust me, I have asked many men their opinion and they often don't prefer this body type—women do. Men tend to want extra body fat and appreciate women who are soft. The media tells us what's beautiful, and then women hold that standard on each other.

What do you see when you picture the feminine? I picture a soft and tender mother-earth type of figure. When I think about femininity I don't picture a woman with bulging biceps, though a woman may have bulging biceps and defined muscles, and that doesn't make her less of a woman. The problem arises when women attempt to abandon their femininity for masculinity. If that occurs, they may find they struggle with their bodies and lives, and they become unbalanced.

The truth is we need a balance of both feminine and masculine energy. There is nothing wrong with wanting to be softer and curvier or hard and defined. Women have physical strength just like any male, and women also have alternate strengths. The feminine energy creates life, nurtures, and shows love and vulnerability. It's the soft, warm hug you need when everything is falling apart. While hitting the punching bag is sometimes needed after a rough day so is curling up in a ball with a stream of tears. One is not better than the other. We need both. And women need to connect to this innate femininity with pride.

This combination of male and female can be viewed in the same way as the macronutrients. We need everything to stay in balance. When it comes to eating, meal planning can help set us up for success with food in this way.

When you are planning your meals, you always want to plan

in sand, not stone, with wiggle room. If planning isn't your thing, however, don't do it. If it truly doesn't feel good and isn't something you want to do the rest of your life, find some other way to live deliciously with food. It just so happens to be more effective for most people because it sets you up for success. Most of my clients say that they eat low-quality food, or more carbohydrates or sugar than feels good to them, when they don't have something planned. When the mind tells the body it's hungry, most bodies will grab whatever is the quickest to quiet the hunger signal—unless they have a plan.

So ask yourself if you want to be someone that plans meals the rest of your life. If you aren't sure, start small. Plan a meal a week and then maybe move toward more. See if that works for your lifestyle or if something else would work better. My personal favorite resource for meal planning is CookSmarts.com. For a very small fee they do the meal planning for you, and you just get the groceries and follow the directions each night.

You also want to look at what your life looks like in your ideal body. Is there meal planning involved or a private chef? Are you dining out often, or are you cooking more? Figure out what your future looks like so you can move toward that.

Lastly, plan to be perfectly imperfect. Skip the gym for a month; eat pizza three days in a row. Whatever it means to be imperfect, do it. I promise it won't kill you. It's healthy. It's called balance.

Most people swing from being "good" to being "bad." They are either eating perfectly planned, healthy meals within their calorie range, or they are binging on pizza and ice cream every day. Therefore, it's only a matter of one meal that can swing them from "good" to "bad." Balance is avoiding both of these extremes. It's allowing ourselves to eat foods that make our bodies feel good most of the time and also eating foods that we want for other reasons.

It's not "bad" to eat cake even though it adds relatively no value to the body. It tastes good. This is a valid reason in itself. If you're hungry for cake, eat it! You will find that your body won't ask for it all that often. However, the only way to get to a place where you don't obsess over cake is to be in balance.

Consider this, too, when you meal plan. Meal planning is not about counting calories or controlling what you eat. It's about ensuring you have access to high-quality food and that you're treating your body correctly.

Since most of you are used to dieting, you are used to having to be perfect when following a meal plan. It is down to the calorie or point. This is misleading. The truth is the formula to tell you how many calories you burn isn't exact. The formula to tell you how many calories are in the food you are eating isn't exact, either. And the process the body uses to break down food and decide whether to burn it or store it is highly influenced by thoughts, beliefs, and emotions.

There is actually something called "the brain-gut connection." Scientists have found a second brain hidden in the walls of the digestive system that they are calling the enteric nervous system (ENS). The role of the ENS is to control digestion, nutrient absorption, and elimination. So while you may think that working that meal plan exactly is your way to control your weight, in reality, you have no control whatsoever. No mind does.

So drop the idea that you can control the body in this manner. You don't really know how many calories you burn, eat, or digest. You don't really know what the body is going to do with those calories. Drop the illusion that you do and just focus on living a balanced, and realistic, lifestyle. One you'll want to live no matter what body you're in.

Questions for Transformation:

1. **What does my body need to switch from fat storing to fat burning?** Where have you told your body you don't have enough? What passion or inspirational idea does it want you to seek?

2. **How can I set myself up for success with food?** Do you need to meal plan? Or use a resource like Cook Smarts, Hello Fresh, etc.? Do you need to hire a private chef or someone to come and prep your food? What would be your ideal scenario with food prep?

3. **What do I need to change in my lifestyle to allow for balance with food, to allow myself to simply eat what sounds good, to notice any reactions, and to adjust accordingly?** What would it take to remove the labels of "good" and "bad," and simply allow food to be food?

Live Fully

Total Body Transformation:

If your only interest is to transform your body, you can literally skip right over this step. You already are on your way.

Total Life Transformation:

This step is for people who desire more than just a smaller body. This is for those of you who want to experience the most incredible lives you can live. In fact, this step can be done completely independently of the others. The steps here help you to create a more balanced and fulfilled life *today*, not once the weight comes off. None of these steps has anything to do with weight. They are simply concepts I have noticed in the minds of people who live extraordinary lives.

Step One: Find Balance

Muscular balance

By now, you might have already experimented with the movements you love and can't live without. If you haven't, now is definitely the time to start! Search for the movements that are going to add value to your life, the ones you're going to love. When you find these loving movements, you are free to eliminate the accountability factor as you are now doing what's natural for your body. If you feel like you have to hold yourself accountable, it isn't the movement for you. In other words, if you have to hold yourself accountable to running, maybe you shouldn't be running.

There is a great deal of debate about what it takes to create new habits. I have found that when someone is properly motivated and aligned, habits can be changed in an instant. There are people who quit smoking cold turkey and never look back. When I started doing yoga, I was addicted after one class; I definitely didn't need 21 or 30 days to establish a habit. I think that when something is a hobby, or you have made a clear decision to change, you don't need to make a habit out of it. It just becomes something you desire to do effortlessly.

If you aren't connecting to any movement, there is a reason for that. Our bodies choose movement naturally unless we really need rest. Therefore, if all movement sounds exhausting, or overwhelming, take some time off and return to it when you are ready.

Eventually, your body will crave movement, but this could take longer for some of you. If you are a workaholic, rest and stillness may be in order to restore balance in your life. If you are high energy, low-heat, slow-moving movements might be right up your alley. If you have been extreme exercising for a long time, your body might not even appreciate movement anymore. It could feel abused.

If you have high stress and high anxiety, your body might feel like it's been exercising all day, fleeing from that lion that's been chasing it. Therefore, you might feel exhausted and like you don't have the energy to move more that day. Honor your body's wishes, but don't allow stress to be your exercise forever. Your body won't fight that battle each and every day.

If you have a job that doesn't require you to sit all day, you might not really need additional exercise. My chiropractor said that after adjusting all day she didn't have the energy to work out. I know this is true because she was very afraid not to work out every day, as she believed it could contribute to weight gain. Therefore, she would drag her tired body on a run anyway. She wasn't enjoying the run. She really wanted to be resting with her family but she didn't think of her work as being active.

If you are one of those people who says, "I swear I am not lazy. I move all day long. I don't know why I have excess weight," then you might need to cut back on your exercise. I don't see any benefit in forcing movement on the days you are running around. On your days off, you might want to do something else. If your job is highly laborious, you might not do anything else. The nice thing is your body will tell you exactly how much movement it requires, so look inward for your muscular-balance principles.

Also be aware that your movement requirements will vary throughout your life. When I had more free time, I went to yoga five to six days a week. This was necessary for me. If I hadn't gone to yoga, all that free time might have triggered my body to fill it with something else when all it really wanted was yoga. Now that I have much less free time, my yoga classes can range from one to four times a week. My body is content with this because I am content with my work. If my work stressed me out and I wasn't enjoying it, I might require more movement.

The amount that equates balance to you really depends on the state of your overall contentment and happiness, as well as the amount of free time you have in your life. When you have lots of free time, I believe your body sees this as an opportunity to get stronger and more flexible. At those times, it seeks more movement to fill your life in healthy ways.

As long as I don't get into a work-only state, my body is happy where it is. If I start to go off balance, it will send me signals to get back in the middle. Those signals could be less movement or more movement. The requirement could be less intense or more. Allow your body to tell you what it wants.

Muscular balance is also making sure that your body has equal flexibility and strength. If you have back pain from tight hamstrings, then you want to make sure you are stretching your hamstrings to be balanced. I highly recommend everyone meets with a trainer at least once to assess where their weakness and strengths are. When you are aware of what muscles to strengthen and lengthen, you can alleviate pain and realign your postural deviations. A good trainer will be able to point all of this out to you after one effective fitness assessment.

Questions for Transformation:

1. **What movements does my body love?** (Keyword BODY)

2. **What movements do I notice only positivity toward?**

3. **Why do I think my body loves them?**

4. **What movements can I try?**

5. **When am I going to try my first movement?** (Be specific)

Pain Balance

Pain, in my opinion, is related to the state of your emotions. If you are experiencing pain, I highly recommend the book *Heal Your Body A-Z* by Louise Hay. This is her area of expertise, and she goes into great detail about how your emotions can trigger pain. This is also the theory that yogis use. When you practice yoga, you will hear the teacher asking you to breathe into the areas of tightness and resistance.

I turn to this theory in my life all the time. Just recently, I got a cold two months in a row. Being someone who almost never gets sick, I was very curious to why this was happening. I had a stuffy nose that wouldn't go away so I looked up what emotion is related to stuffy nose in Hay's book, and it said not recognizing self worth. The next day I had a call with my coach and after she read my prep form she said, "I feel like you are not recognizing your self worth." I was blown away! I made it a point to focus on this topic, and the stuffy nose went away instantly.

I know what works for one doesn't work for all. There are people who have visited the healer, chiropractor, or masseuse, and it hasn't worked for them. But I also know that when we do have physical ailments and diseases, it's a valid excuse to not step up in life. A person in pain might say, "I can't do that, I have too much pain" or "I shouldn't move, I have too much pain." It's an easy, valid excuse. It's a way to settle. Therefore, I believe it's important to approach pain from various different aspects. Think about pain from the mental/emotional/spiritual aspect, as well as the physical.

Another approach to pain balance is utilizing strategic movements. We can use yoga to strengthen muscles that are weak, stretch, and/or align the spine. We also can choose a holistic healer like a chiropractor, masseuse, acupuncturist, etc. to help. In whatever method you choose, be picky! Find the one that works for you, and don't settle.

What I notice with pain is that people really settle in their lives. They switch from living to surviving, moving just to get through the day. When we experience chronic pain, then we can assume it's part of our lives forever. The truth is that pain is an opportunity to pay attention. Be grateful for pain because it's giving you a message from your body. Honor its information. Be invested and committed to solutions. Stay in a creative, problem-solving state.

Use medication or pharmaceutical procedures to alleviate symptoms so that you can search for a cause and a long-term solution to your pain. Using drugs is a fast and easy way to get rid of pain, but we get pain for a reason. It's communication. So stay curious throughout the process, instead of being angry or down because you are experiencing it. Figure out what you can learn from it.

For example, if you have back pain, you may learn that you simply need to make it a practice to stretch daily. This can help you feel better in more ways than one if you love stretching for peace and happiness. Whatever is needed to find symptom alleviation and the cause, don't stop until you find the answer. Visit 400 doctors until you find the solution for you if needed. Go to several types of healers—a traditional doctor, a holistic doctor, etc. Find the one that fits your needs.

Don't settle for pain or just getting through life. You cannot live fully when you are in pain every single day.

Questions for Transformation:

1. **How am I going to begin living my life and not just getting through it?**

2. **What is my first step toward less pain?**

Energy Balance

Energy balance is all about balancing work, play, and rest. A full life needs all three, though we often are not taught that from society. Instead, we are taught that we have to work hard, go to school, get good grades to get into college, and then get a good job to succeed.

You are not a stranger to the depiction of the work-a-holic dad who misses his son's baseball game ... again. Or the mom who chooses to work 80 hours a week instead of stay at home with her kids, and therefore has a limited relationship with her children.

These made-for-movie scenarios may be slightly exaggerated, but the message behind them is valid. We live in a society that places high value on work, a small value on play (work hard, play hard), and relatively zero value on rest (I'll sleep when I'm dead).

While these themes may not have been formally discussed with you, they are present where we live and hard to ignore.

Let's say you just lost 100 pounds. Naturally, each person you see is going to make a comment about how fantastic you look followed up by, "How did you do it?" There are two answers you might give, and I want you to pay careful attention to your reactions to each.

Answer one:

"I decided to go on a low-calorie diet by having a shake for breakfast every morning, a salad for lunch, and then a dinner of steamed vegetables and a lean protein. I made sure I kept all treats out of the house, and I let myself have one cheat day per week on Sunday when I could have whatever I wanted. Every day after work, I went to the gym to a high-intensity boot camp and on the weekends I either ran, walked, or rode my bike. It took a lot of willpower to turn down food when I was around it, but I stayed strong for six months and lost 100 pounds. It was incredibly difficult to stick to this plan but I was highly motivated and made it a priority. The worst was social events, and so after a couple I simply stayed away and just tried to stay busy other ways so I didn't think about food. If I wanted to eat, I would turn on an exercise DVD or busy my hands some other way."

Answer two:

"I decided to learn how to eat when I was hungry and stop when I was full. Once I stopped dieting, it happened really easily and took relatively no effort at all. I worked out when I felt like it and did lower intensity exercises because my body feels best with those. I honestly didn't put much thought at all into losing weight and really just focused on things that were fun. I went to more social events, planned more adventures, and got more creative. I enjoyed my time more and rested a lot more. I added time for yoga and relaxation, and even just spent some days lying around reading. Honestly, the hardest part was just staying present but the losing weight part wasn't hard at all."

Most people would say that answer two sounds really great, but that there is a lot more value in answer one. Answer one shows a dedicated, hard-working individual that stuck to her plan and exercised willpower like crazy. Most people would give accolades, praise, and even feel envious that they couldn't stick with a plan for six months. And most people would assume that answer two was a fluke, a lucky break, and would most likely never work for them.

Why do we think this way?

Most people say they are tired of weight loss and maintenance being so hard, yet when they're offered a solution that doesn't include the typical type of hard work, they immediately discount it. They don't see the value in it, and they don't feel it will work.

The problem is the value of hard work has taken over our society and caused us to swing massively out of balance.

The best way to create balance is to create boundaries. You need a certain amount of work, play, and rest to thrive in your life, and you intuitively know how much of each. Your body gives you cues when it needs more work. It may crave growth, challenge, passion, or inspiration. If you are needing more fun, you will find yourself filling time with numbing activities like television, technology, or binge eating. And if you need more rest, your body may experience pain, sickness, or just exhaustion. These are examples from my life. It may look different for you, but your body will definitely send you cues to let you know you are out of balance.

When I tried to lose weight without success, I was addicted to working hard at it. I figured if I was going to have excess weight, I had to verify my efforts to the world. As long as I worked super hard at losing weight every single day I could declare to the world that I was trying. I had moments in which I gave up entirely, but it wasn't long before I shamed myself back into working hard, even without any glimmer of success.

When I lost weight while injured on the couch, it felt like a fluke. At first I didn't believe it. And then, even when it was confirmed, I went right back to my work-hard attitude to remove the rest of the weight. It wasn't until I refocused on fulfilling my needs, balancing my life, and sticking to my boundaries that the rest of the weight actually came off, though.

I carried the same mistake into my business. Each day, I worked super hard to grow my business, to make more money, to show that I was successful. And when it didn't work (and it never did), I worked harder so that I could tell the world that I was trying. I couldn't very well sit on the couch watching TV all day and then complain I wasn't making money. So I had to keep working hard to distract from the imbalances I was, once again, creating in my life.

Until, that is, I got honest with myself. The truth was I didn't want to work so hard that I couldn't go on vacation and do yoga. I didn't want to work on the weekends and never be able to leave an email unanswered. I wanted to be able to unplug from my business and be with my family. I wanted to feel as though I had more of a life than just someone who worked and made money. And so it wasn't until I created that type of business that it started to succeed.

Is your life balanced? Are you working more than you are playing? Do you value hard work so much that you believe it's the only way you can be successful?

You only have one life to live in this body. Do you want to work really hard until age 65 and then retire? Or do you want to work somewhat hard and play a lot now?

If you are working too hard, how can you create boundaries to create more balance in your life? You may need to delegate more or have a tough conversation with a boss or with yourself. You may need to hire a mentor who has mastered the art of success in business without working 100 hours per week.

If you are not getting enough rest, start with your quality of sleep. Talk with a professional about your problems with sleep and try out different solutions until you find the one for you. When you are resting and relaxing, actually rest and relax. This means removing stimulation and becoming present, not numbing out or feeling stressed about what you should be doing instead.

If you aren't getting enough play, it's time to have some fun. Write down all the things you do for fun and all the things you'd like to try. Plan events throughout the month, like a monthly happy hour or a craft day with friends. Join a low-key softball league to have some fun and get some activity. Turn off the television, put your phone on silent, and ask yourself, "What do I want to do or what do I need?"

Take personal health days. If things are getting stressful and crazy, and you are working too hard, you will get out of balance. If you don't take that time for yourself to fulfill your needs you will continue to spiral out of balance. This is when catastrophic events may occur in an attempt to restore some balance in your life.

Work, play, and rest are all equally important. Work gives us purpose and a sense of accomplishment. Play gives us value and fun. Rest gives us the ability to do all of it all over again with full energy. Therefore, it is important that you are honest with yourself about what is serving you at all times.

This energy balance also means that you live out of a place

of choice. This means you can say with full conviction, "I choose to be relaxed today." "I choose to yell at the traffic." "I choose to make less money."

If you are looking at that less-money statement and asking who in her right mind would choose less money, I've got news for you, it could be you. If a family member left you 10 million dollars at the top of the tallest mountain and all you had to do was climb the mountain and it was yours, would you do it? It would be hard, cold, and probably sheer agony. So is that money worth sacrificing your well-being? Is it worth risking the cold and pain to get 10 million dollars? Some of you will say "yes," and some will say, "no way!" The question is: Is it worth it?

Questions for Transformation:

1. **If I could wave a magic wand, what would my life look like?** Write out the whole story of what your dream life would be.

2. **Am I honoring my wishes for rest and play versus work, according to my new story?**

Step Two: Meditate

Meditation has been the key to peace and happiness in my life. It is a forced way to slow down. If you know that you need to slow down in life, what better way than to take two minutes to close your eyes?

Meditation beneficially changes the brain. This has been proven by science. In the past, scientists didn't realize that the brain was able to change so dramatically. Now, however, studies have shown that meditation can increase cortical thickness, density of grey matter, connectivity of white matter, and network connectivity.

On a practical level, meditation also helps to reduce stress, improve wellbeing, and ultimately re-wire the brain. A study done in 2016 compared a group of meditators to a group of non-meditators. While all the participants stated they felt better at the end of the day, only the mediators showed changes in the brain scan. These changes have been linked to less inflammation and less stress.

While meditating is perceived as a way to clear the mind, you may feel that as soon as you close your eyes every thought comes rushing through. It might feel impossible to clear your mind, but don't give up. The intrusive thoughts will lessen with practice, and your mind will quiet faster and faster each time. Don't focus on getting rid of your thoughts, just watch them go by, and don't follow them. Let them roam through your head.

When you're first starting out, you may think, *Wow I'm hungry!* Normally, when you have this thought you begin to think about what you want to eat, where you want to eat, etc. This triggers a longer thought process. When you are meditating, however, you want to acknowledge the thought, and then tell it you will think about it when you are done with your meditation.

Meditation also connects mind, body, and sprit. Yoga is a preparation for mediation. The asanas are just postures and only take up one limb of yoga. Part of yoga is the way we live, breathe, and move, but the ultimate goal is to meditate. The movement of yoga is to prepare the body for the end, when we rest in corpse pose.

It is my belief that meditation is the best way to lose weight. The more time you spend in the parasympathetic branch of the nervous system, the more relaxed you feel, which is the optimal state for weight loss. Meditation helps you connect to your body. When you are connected to your body, you trigger true, long-lasting weight loss.

The more you meditate, and find that clear mind, the more you can ask your subconscious the tough questions. Questions that, if you had the answers to, could change your life for the better. Questions like, "Why am I lacking self worth?

What does my body need in order to lose weight? Why am I struggling?" It can be difficult to adopt new beliefs, but working toward clearing the mind allows true, total transformation to happen.

If you have never used meditation or you aren't sure how to begin, use guided meditations! If you are by yourself it will keep you focused. These meditations will walk you through different peaceful scenarios. And, if you fall asleep, it's ok! It's all a journey! My favorite guided meditations are from MeditationOasis.com.

Questions for Transformation:

How can I add a meditation practice into my life? Do you need to download guided meditations? Do you need to meditate first thing in the morning or right before bed? Do you need to set a timer on your phone to stop and take deep breaths?

Conclusion

You wake up with the sun on your face. With a full body stretch and a yawn, you glance out the window to see the beauty that lies outside. It's always been there, you realize, but now it's just more obvious. You reach over to your tablet and hit play on your favorite meditation.

In the background, you hear your son talking to himself and playing with his toys in his bedroom. You think about giving him a hug and a kiss right after you finish your meditation, but this is your time to come into your body and breathe deeply into the most authentic version of you. When your meditation is done, you carefully step out of bed. On the way out the door toward your son's room, you smile.

I feel really good, you think. And just when you think you couldn't be any happier, you open the door to see the smiling face of your son.

After saying good morning, you make your way to the kitchen to prepare breakfast for yourself and your son. You carefully crack the eggs into the pan, add salt and pepper, and decide that sourdough bread sounds delicious with your eggs this morning. For a moment, old programming comes back and reminds you that "bread is bad," which you quickly dismiss, remembering that bread is just bread. It's not bad or good. And you are hungry, which means eating—and eating what sounds good to you—is a good thing.

You set the food down in front of your son and reach down to take your first bite thinking that life can't get any more blissful. Your thoughts of gratitude are interrupted by the feeling of warm, oily butter sliding down the side of your face. In the past, your son throwing his food would have been enough to set off your entire day. But now, you wipe your face, take three deep breaths, and continue eating your carefully prepared breakfast.

After breakfast, you begin to get ready for your day while your son plays with his toys. You look through your closet, deciding what would feel amazing on your body today. Your closet is full of clothes you adore, and it took you a while to build a wardrobe that suits you so perfectly. Even in your lighter, more ideal body, you still have rolls and dimples, but with determination and focus you found clothes at the store that were flattering on your very real, but ideal, body.

You feel confident as you get dressed, but not because you tricked your body into getting smaller through force, deprivation, or extreme dieting. You feel confident because you truly feel good. You haven't overeaten in months. Your binge eating has completely disappeared, and you look forward with excitement to moving your body each day. You also cherish your moments of rest and relaxation, and you love to play and be silly with your husband and son.

You no longer stare wistfully as they eat their Cheetos together and laugh uncontrollably. Now, some days, you join them, eating and laughing, matching Cheetos dust on all your faces. Other days, you find you're not hungry and Cheetos don't sound good to you so you effortlessly say no with a smile and a sense of fulfillment.

Your body is far from perfect, but it's your body. You love it and appreciate it. It's a body that has taken you to thousands of places without complaining most of the time. It contains the power of creation, whether it has created human life or a brilliant piece of art. It effortlessly takes care of everything on the inside that keeps you alive so you can focus on laughing, playing, creating, and being a part of the world you live in.

Your body, in turn, appreciates being taken care of and rewards you as much as it can. It also communicates to you through body symptoms such as pain, illness, disease, and yes, sometimes a snug pair of pants. But these aren't seen as alarm bells for panic; they are seen as the beginning of a conversation between your body and you.

Instead of getting frustrated and angry when you get these messages, you get curious and ask the body what it needs. You intuitively take a scan of what could make your life even better, and immediately act to fulfill this. The body responds to your intentional and clear actions by loosening the waistline of your pants once again.

After a last-minute glance in the mirror to make sure your clothes and hair are in place, you snuggle your son and get ready to head off to daycare. With hugs and kisses, you say your goodbyes as you then calmly leave to head out to conquer your day. Some days are for focused and intense work. Some days, you choose to play a little.

Overall your days feel light and free, but you don't expect every day to be perfect. You realize that life is messy, bumpy, and anything but linear. You allow for stressors and do your best to breathe through them. You mediate more and work less when it's necessary. You take time for you, and you make time for the people that matter most.

You turn your phone on silent when you need peace, even leaving it in a different room at times. You are present for the people you need and for yourself. You realize the importance in taking breaks from technology, television, and stimulation in general. You find balance in disconnecting from the external and reconnecting with the internal.

Food is now something you enjoy immensely, but it isn't a major focus. At the end of the day, it's just food. Your time and energy are spent engaging in many more passionate and pleasurable activities than just food. You do, however, love to give food attention, love, and care when hunger strikes, and you do your best to stay prepared with nutritious food and meals so you can be better prepared to eat the way you truly desire to eat.

Movement is something you do for fun, to challenge your body and because it feels good. It's never forced, and there are even times you skip it for a duration of time. But you effortlessly come back to it time and time again. You honor your desires, and do what your body finds exciting and pleasurable. Yoga was your passion for several months. Now you are feeling a desire to try out a dance class, and you're searching for the perfect class for you.

When you walk into the store later that day to grab some food for the week you see a woman carefully investigating a loaf of bread. You notice her cart is full of diet meals and low-calorie snacks, and it is void of anything with sugar. You see the agony on her face as she argues with herself about purchasing this loaf of bread. Maybe bread is to her what potato chips were for you, something that cannot be trusted in the house.

Seeing this woman reminds you how far you have come. Without comparing or judging her, you understand completely how she feels. Her life was your life for so long. But now, it's different. While glancing at labels to check ingredients is still important to you, the agony around food is gone. And for this, you are forever grateful.

You also feel at peace in your body. This peace doesn't feel temporary or fleeing. It feels permanent and fixed. You have mastered the art of living in a body you love, even without it being perfect. You don't look like the cover of a magazine but you are clear this body is ideal for you. Even more importantly, your life is ideal. It has bumps and blips, but it's your life, and you feel lucky to have it. It's full, joyous, and delicious.

As you walk out of the grocery store door with your bags, the late afternoon sun warms your face. You look up and smile.

Sincerely,

Michelle

P.S. I hope you enjoyed this book! Remember, I am available to walk the journey with you. I've been where you are, and I've come out the other side. I've also helped countless others walk the path before you. If you want maximum support and human-to-human contact, simply fill out an application at totalbodyhealthsolutions.com/getsupport.

If you qualify, I will personally get on the phone with you and help guide you through this process.

And, hey, if you enjoy my books, please share them with loved ones, and review them!

The Weight Loss Shift: Be More, Weigh Less

The Chakra Secret: What Your Body Is Telling You

Have Your Cake and Be Happy, Too: A Joyful Approach to Weight Loss

Women Will Save the World

About Michelle Hastie

Michelle Hastie is a weight loss coach and author with expertise in personal training, food psychology, neuro-linguistic programming, and yoga. Through her company, Total Body Health Solutions, she is blessed with the gift of helping individuals eat when they are hungry, stop when they are full, and move their bodies without force. She has a master's degree in human behavior and is pursuing a doctorate in health psychology to further promote the art and science of weight loss through mind-body awareness.

Hastie helps people learn to love their bodies and transform their lives through her Absolute Love Publishing books, *The Weight Loss Shift: Be More, Weigh Less*; *The Chakra Secret: What Your Body Is Telling You*; and *Have Your Cake and Be Happy, Too: A Joyful Approach to Weight Loss*. She also is a contributor to the Amazon category bestseller *Women Will Save the World*.

Did you enjoy this book?

Please consider leaving a brief review on Amazon for Michelle Hastie's books, inlcuding *The Weight Loss Shift: Be More, Weigh Less*; *The Chakra Secret: What Your Body Is Telling You*; *Have Your Cake and Be Happy, Too: A Joyful Approach to Weight Loss*; and *Women Will Save the World*.

Would you like to know about the latest Absolute Love Publishing releases? Join our newsletter on our website home page: www.absolutelovepublishing.com.

About Absolute Love Publishing

Absolute Love Publishing is an independent book publisher devoted to creating and publishing books that promote goodness in the world.

www.absolutelovepublishing.com

Books by Absolute Love Publishing

Adult Fiction and Non-Fiction Books

The Chakra Secret: What Your Body Is Telling You, a min-e-book™ by Michelle Hastie
Do you believe there may be more to the body than meets the eye? Have you wondered why you run into the same physical issues over and over again? Maybe you are dealing with dis-eases or ailments and are ready to treat more than just the symptoms. Or perhaps you've simply wondered why you gain weight in your midsection while your friend gains weight in her hips? Get ready to understand how powerful energy centers in your body communicate messages from beyond the physical. Discover the root, energetic problems that are causing imbalances, and harness a universal power to create drastic changes in your happiness, your well-being, and your body with *The Chakra Secret: What Your Body Is Telling You*, a min-e-book™.

Finding Happiness with Migraines: a Do It Yourself Guide, a min-e-book™ by Sarah Hackley
Do you have monthly, weekly, or even daily migraines? Do you feel lonely or isolated, or like you are constantly worrying about the next impending migraine attack? Is the weight of living with migraine disease dampening your enjoyment of the "now"? Experience the happiness you crave with *Finding Happiness with Migraines: a Do It Yourself Guide*, a min-e-book™ by Sarah Hackley.

Discover how you can take charge of your body, your mind, your emotions, and your health by practicing simple, achievable steps that create a daily life filled with more joy, appreciation, and confidence. Sarah's Five Steps to Finding

Happiness with Migraines provide an actionable path to a new, happier way of living with migraine disease. A few of the tools you'll learn: which yoga poses can help with a migraine attack, why you should throw away your daily migraine journal, how do-it-yourself therapy can create positive change, and techniques to connect with your body and intuition.

Have Your Cake and Be Happy, Too: A Joyful Approach to Weight Loss by Michelle Hastie

Have you tried every weight loss trick and diet out there only to still feel stuck with unwanted body fat? Are you ready to live joyfully and fully, in a body that stores only the amount of fat it needs? Then this book is for you.

In *Have Your Cake and Be Happy, Too: A Joyful Approach to Weight Loss*, author Michelle Hastie uses her own research into nutrition and the psychology of weight loss to help you uncover the mindset you need to transition from fat storing to fat burning, without overly fancy or external tactics. No more strict regimens or unfulfilling meals. Just strong body awareness, deep mind-body connection, and positive results. Don't change your diet or your exercise routine. Instead, pick up this book, and change your life.

Love Like God: Embracing Unconditional Love

In this groundbreaking compilation, well-known individuals from across the globe share stories of how they learned to release the conditions that block absolute love. Along with the insights of bestselling author Caroline A. Shearer, readers will be reminded of their natural state of love and will begin to envision a world without fear or judgement or pain. Along with Shearer's reflections and affirmations, experts, musicians, authors, professional athletes, and others shed light on the universal experiences of journeying the path of unconditional love.

Love Like God Companion Book

You've read the love-expanding essays from the luminaries of *Love Like God*. Now, take your love steps further with the *Love Like God Companion Book*. The Companion provides a positive, actionable pathway into a state of absolute love, enabling readers to further open their hearts at a pace that matches their experiences. This book features an expanded introduction, the Thoughts and Affirmations from *Love Like God*, plus all new "Love in Action Steps."

Preparing to Fly: Financial Freedom from Domestic Abuse by Sarah Hackley

Are financial worries keeping you stuck in an abusive or unhealthy relationship? Do you want to break free but don't know how to make it work financially? Take charge with *Preparing to Fly*, a personal finance book for women who want to escape the relationships that are holding them back.

Drawing on personal experiences and nearly a decade of financial expertise, Sarah Hackley walks readers step-by-step through empowering plans and tools: Learn how much money it will take to leave and how much you'll need to live on your own. Change the way you think about money to promote your independence. Bring control of your life back to where it belongs—with you. Break free and live in your own power, with *Preparing to Fly*. Additional tips for women with children, married women, pregnant women, the chronically ill, and more!

The Weight Loss Shift: Be More, Weigh Less by Michelle Hastie

The Weight Loss Shift: Be More, Weigh Less by Michelle Hastie helps those searching for their ideal bodies shift into a higher way of being, inviting the lasting weight they want—along with the life of their dreams! Skip the diets and the gimmicks, *The Weight Loss Shift* is a permanent weight loss solution. Based on science, psychology, and spirituality, Hastie helps readers discover their ideal way of being through detailed instructions and exercises, and then helps readers transform to living a life free from worry about weight—forever!

Would you like to love your body at any weight? Would you like to filter through others' body expectations to discover your own? Would you like to live at your ideal weight naturally, effortlessly, and happily? Then make the shift with *The Weight Loss Shift: Be More, Weigh Less*!

Where Is the Gift? Discovering the Blessing in Every Situation, a min-e-book™ by Caroline A. Shearer

Inside every challenge is a beautiful blessing waiting for us to unwrap it. All it takes is our choice to learn the lesson of the challenge! Are you in a situation that is challenging you? Are you struggling with finding the perfect blessing the universe is holding for you? This min-e-book™ will help you unwrap your blessings with more ease and grace, trust in the perfect manifestation of your life's challenges, and move through life with the smooth path your higher self intended. Make the choice: unwrap your gift today!

Women Will Save the World

Leading women across the nation celebrate the feminine nature through stories of collaboration, creativity, intuition, nurturing, strength, trailblazing, and wisdom in *Women Will Save the World*. Inspired by a quote from the Dalai Lama, bestselling author and Absolute Love Publishing Founder Caroline A. Shearer brings these inherent feminine qualities to the forefront, inviting a discussion of the impact women have on humanity and initiating the question: Will women save the world?

The Adventures of a Lightworker Series by Caroline A. Shearer

Dead End Date
Dead End Date is the first book in a metaphysical series about a woman's crusade to teach the world about love, one mystery and personal hang-up at a time. In a Bridget Jones meets New Age-style, *Dead End Date* introduces readers to Faith, a young woman whose dating disasters and personal angst have separated her from the reason she's on Earth. When she receives the shocking news that she is a lightworker and has one year to fulfill her life purpose, Faith embarks on her mission with zeal, tackling problems big and small—including the death of her blind date. Working with angels and psychic abilities and even the murder victim himself, Faith dives headfirst into a personal journey that will transform all those around her and, eventually, all those around the world.

The Raise Your Vibration Series by Caroline A. Shearer

Raise Your Vibration: Tips and Tools for a High-Frequency Life, a min-e-book™
Presenting mind-opening concepts and tips, *Raise Your Vibration: Tips and Tools for a High-Frequency Life*, a min-e-book™, opens the doorway to your highest and greatest good! This min-e-book™ demonstrates how every thought and every action affect our level of attraction, enabling us to attain what we truly want in life.

As beings of energy that give off and respond to vibration, it's important we understand the clarity, fullness, and happiness that come from living at a higher frequency. Divided into categories of mind, body, and spirit/soul, readers will learn practical steps they immediately can put into practice to resonate at a higher vibration and to further evolve their souls. A must-read primer for a higher existence! Are you ready for a high-frequency life?

Raise Your Financial Vibration: Tips and Tools to Embrace Your Infinite Spiritual Abundance, a min-e-book™

Are you ready to release the mind dramas that hold you back from your infinite spiritual abundance? Are you ready for a high-frequency financial life? Allow, embrace, and enjoy your infinite spiritual abundance and financial wealth today!

Absolute Love Publishing Creator Caroline A. Shearer explores simple steps and shifts in mindset that will help you receive the abundance you desire in *Raise Your Financial Vibration: Tips and Tools to Embrace Your Infinite Spiritual Abundance*, a min-e-book™. Learn how to release blocks to financial abundance, create thought patterns that will help you achieve a more desirable financial reality, and fully step into an abundant lifestyle by discovering the art of being abundant.

Raise Your Verbal Vibration: Create the Life You Want with Law of Attraction Language, a min-e-book™

Are the words you speak bringing you closer to the life you want? Or are your word choices inadvertently creating more difficulties? Discover words and phrases that are part of the Language of Light in Absolute Love Publishing Creator Caroline A. Shearer's latest in the Raise Your Vibration min-e-book™ series: *Raise Your Verbal Vibration: Create the Life You Want with Law of Attraction Language.* Learn what common phrases and words may be holding you back, and utilize a list of high-vibration words that you can begin to incorporate into your vocabulary. Increase your verbal vibration today with this compelling addition to the Raise Your Vibration series!

Young Adult and Children's Books

Dear One, Be Kind by Jennifer Farnham

This beautiful children's book takes young children on a journey of harmony and empathy. Using rhyme and age-appropriate language and imagery, *Dear One, Be Kind* illustrates how children can embrace feelings of kindness and love for everyone they meet, even when others are seemingly hurtful. By revealing the unseen message behind common childhood experiences, the concept of empathy is introduced, along with a gentle knowledge of our interconnectedness and the belief that, through kindness, children have the power to change their world. Magically illustrated with a soothing and positive message, this book is a joy for children and parents alike!

The Adima Chronicles by Steve Schatz

Adima Rising

For millennia, the evil Kroledutz have fed on the essence of humans and clashed in secret with the Adima, the light weavers of the universe. Now, with the balance of power shifting toward darkness, time is running out. Guided by a timeless Native American spirit, four teenagers from a small New Mexico town discover they have one month to awaken their inner power and save the world.

Rory, Tima, Billy, and James must solve four ancient challenges by the next full moon to awaken a mystical portal and become Adima. If they fail, the last threads of light will dissolve, and the universe will be lost forever. Can they put aside their fears and discover their true natures before it's too late?

Adima Returning

The Sacred Cliff is crumbling and with it the Adima way of life! Weakened by the absence of their beloved friend

James, Rory, Tima, and Billy must battle time and unseen forces to unite the greatest powers of all dimensions in one goal. They must move the Sacred Cliff before it traps all Adima on Earth—and apart from the primal energy of the Spheres—forever!

Aided by a surprising and timeless maiden, the three light-weaving teens travel across the planes of existence to gain help from the magical creatures who guard the Adima's most powerful objects, the Olohos. There is only one path to success: convince the guardians to help. Fail and the Cliff dissolves, destroying the once-eternal Spheres and the interdimensional light weavers known as Adima.

Like the exciting adventures of *Adima Rising*, the second spellbinding book of The Adima Chronicles, *Adima Returning*, will have your senses reeling right up until its across-worlds climax. Will conscious creation and the bonds of friendship be enough to fight off destructive forces and save the world once again?

The Soul Sight Mysteries by Janet McLaughlin

Haunted Echo
Sun, fun, toes in the sand, and daydreams about her boyfriend back home. That's what teen psychic Zoey Christopher expects for her spring break on an exotic island. But from the moment she steps foot onto her best friend Becca's property, Zoey realizes the island has other plans: chilling drum beats, a shadowy ghost, and a mysterious voodoo doll.

Zoey has always seen visions of the future, but when she arrives at St. Anthony's Island to vacation among the jet set, she has her first encounter with a bona fide ghost. Forced to uncover the secret behind the girl's untimely death, Zoey quickly realizes that trying to solve the case will thrust her into mortal danger—and into the arms of a budding crush.

Can Zoey put the tormented spirit's soul to rest without her own wild emotions haunting her?

Fireworks

Dreams aren't real. Psychic teen Zoey Christopher knows the difference between dreams and visions better than anyone, but ever since she and her best friend returned from spring vacation, Zoey's dreams have been warning her that Becca is in danger. But a dream isn't a vision—right?

Besides, Zoey has other things to worry about, like the new, cute boy in school. Dan obviously has something to hide, and he won't leave Zoey alone—even when it causes major problems with Josh, Zoey's boyfriend. Is it possible he knows her secret?

Then, one night, Becca doesn't answer any of Zoey's texts or calls. She doesn't answer the next morning either. When Zoey's worst fears come true, her only choice is to turn to Dan, whom she discovers has a gift different from her own but just as powerful. Is it fate? Will using their gifts together help them save Becca, or will the darkness win?

Discover what's real and what's just a dream in *Fireworks*, book two of the Soul Sight Mysteries!

• • •

Connect with us and learn more about our books and upcoming releases at AbsoluteLovePublishing.com.